KUB in Urology Practice

Mr. Jorge Clavijo-Eisele, FEBU.

Editor: Mr Jorge Clavijo-Eisele, MD, FEBU.

Assisted by: Mr Raja Marimuthu MRCS.

Contributors: Mr Graham Watson FRCS, Mr Prateek Verma FRCS, Mr William Lawrence FRCS, Mr Peter Rimington FRCS.

Director of publications and Project manager: Mr J. Clavijo-Eisele.

Printer: CreateSpace. North Charleston, SC. USA.

Publisher: Urology Solutions Publishing.

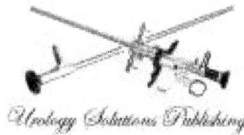

Urology Solutions Publishing

Every effort has been made to contact copyright holders and to ensure that all the information presented is correct. Some of the facts in this volume may be subject to debate or dispute. If proper copyright acknowledgment has not been made, or for clarifications and corrections, please contact the publishers and we will correct the information.

ISBN: 978-0-9931760-1-2

DEDICATION

To my family.

To the Urology team at Eastbourne DGH of 2004.

CONTENTS

DEDICATION iii

CONTENTS i

INTRODUCTION 1

CHAPTER 1. INDICATIONS OF A KUB. 7

CHAPTER 2. TECHNIQUE. 9

CHAPTER 3. FILM ANALYSIS. 11

CHAPTER 4. ABNORMAL FINDINGS. 25

CHAPTER 5. CAVEATS. 67

CHAPTER 6. LATERAL AND OBLIQUE FILMS. 69

AFTERWORD. 73

GLOSSARY. 75

INDEX. 77

INTRODUCTION.

If you want to be sleek and expeditious managing Urology patients, you need imaging tools. A KUB X-ray is one of the oldest, least invasive and perfectly useful ones.

This book will hopefully help you to improve the use of a KUB, and explain how the study helps in problem solution and decision making.

Mr J. Clavijo

KUB in Urology Practice

Mr J. Clavijo

4

"To gain freedom is to gain simplicity."

Joan Miró i Ferrà.

Mr J. Clavijo

CHAPTER 1. INDICATIONS OF A KUB.

This simple radiological study can be the first step of an IVU or a standalone examination. It implies the exposure of the patient's abdomen and pelvis, with mild angulation, to a single dose of X rays that will produce a plain film. The radiation dose is in average 0.664 rem[1].

In a KUB, as in an Abdominal XR or Chest XR one can differentiate images in a scale of greys.

The information provided by the study will be enough to make decisions and in some cases, to decide on patient management or follow up.

The film is aimed to provide information on the urinary tract and also on abdominal contents and osteo-muscular structures.

Like any other examination, a KUB should be requested to answer a specific clinical question[2]. It is critical to remember that having it done implies the exposure (although low) to cumulative ionizing radiation. Ionizing radiation has permanent effects on biological tissues, so the trade-off has to be balanced and discussed with the patient whenever possible, in an adequate way. The choice and frequency of subsequent imaging ought to be guided by the clinical course[3].

Usual indications:
- Renal colic[4]
- Follow up of radio-opaque renal stones[5]
- Acute abdomen
- Acute flank pain[6]
- Positioning control of indwelling devices (JJ stents, etc.)
- Assessing radiopaque foreign bodies

Contraindications:
- Pregnancy
- Known radio-lucent stones

[1] Bush WH, Jones D, Gibbons RP. Radiation dose to patient and personnel during extracorporeal shock wave lithotripsy. J Urol. 1987 Oct; 138(4):716-9.

[2] Dyer RB, Chen MY, Zagoria RJ. Intravenous urography: technique and interpretation. Radiographics. 2001 Jul-Aug; 21(4):799-821.

[3] Johri N, Cooper B, Robertson W, Choong S, Rickards D, Unwin R. An update and practical guide to renal stone management. Nephron Clin Pract. 2010; 116(3):c159-71.

[4] Henderson SO, Hoffner RJ, Aragona JL, Groth DE, Esekogwu VI, Chan D. Bedside emergency department ultrasonography plus radiography of the kidneys, ureters, and bladder vs intravenous pyelography in the evaluation of suspected ureteral colic. Acad Emerg Med 1998; 5:666-671

[5] Assi Z, Platt JF, Francis IR, Cohan RH, Korobkin M. Sensitivity of CT scout radiography and abdominal radiography for revealing ureteral calculi on helical CT: implications for radiologic follow-up. AJR Am J Roentgenol. 2000 Aug; 175(2):333-7.

[6] Svedstrom E, Alanen A, Nurmi M. Radiologic diagnosis of renal colic: the role of plain film, excretory urography and sonography. Eur J Radiol 1990; 11:180-183.

CHAPTER 2. TECHNIQUE.

From the technical point of view the film must include the lower two ribs and the whole pubic symphysis and it must be properly centred.

It should be adequately penetrated so that the different shadows of grey will give the most possible information. These should allow to properly differentiate the various soft tissues that make up the region (kidney, liver shadow, spleen, and psoas) and the skeleton.

Prior to exposure the patient must remove all clothes and personal piercings that may interfere with the study. Shadows originating from the body surface (bandages, clothes, buttons, and buckles) should be avoided. Any piece of radiation absorbing material (metal in particular) will produce a change to the image and consequent degradation of the information obtainable.

The kidney, ureter, bladder (KUB) radiograph is an indispensable part of the sequence of an IVU. This image should be obtained with the appropriate technique (65–75 kV, high milliamperage -30 to 40 mAs-, and short exposure time) to maximize inherent soft-tissue contrast and optimize visualization of calcium-containing lesions.

The patient should void immediately prior to undergoing this examination, and have all jewellery removed or moved away from the examination area. Then lie on the back on the radiology table. There should be no rotation of the shoulder or pelvis. The patient's arms must be at the sides and away from the body.

A gonadal shield can be used on males. In this case the upper edge of the shield should be below the pubic symphysis protecting the testicles.

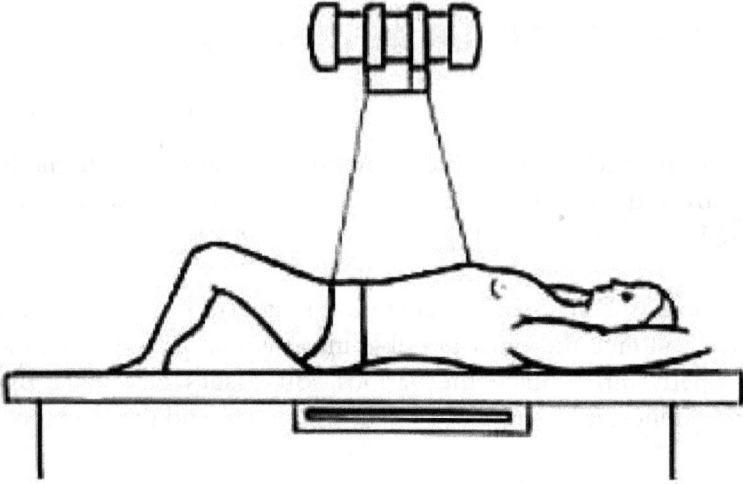

Two radiographs may be needed if the patient is tall or obese. The X ray exposure is made during expiration. This moves the diaphragm to its superior position and results in better visualization of the abdominal contents.

The radiograph is usually performed in the supine position, but if the patient problems suggests pneumoperitoneum, urinary extravasation etc., additional shots must be made in different decubitus or standing.

CHAPTER 3. FILM ANALYSIS.

"You won't see it if you don't know what to look for."

To analyse the film the following approach will help you to know what to look for:

1. Osteo-muscular system:

a.   Bones.

Look for metal sutures, screws and nails that indicate previous treatments, osteoblastic (whiter) and osteolythic (darker) metastasis and fractures, particularly in the axial skeleton. Shadows of the costal cartilages and of the transverse processes of the lumbar vertebrae (calcified costal cartilages).

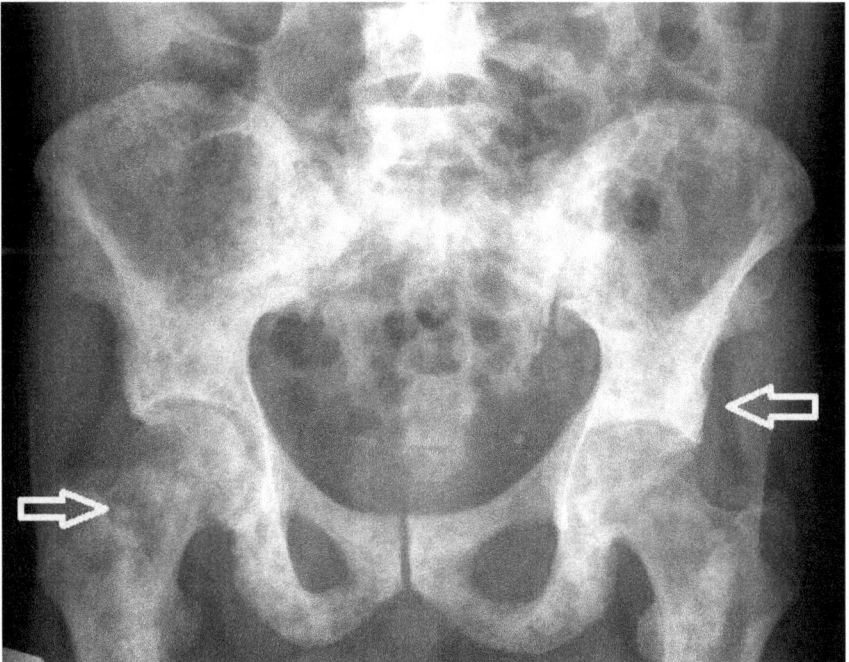

Multiple osteoblastic (radio-opaque) metastasis from prostate cancer.

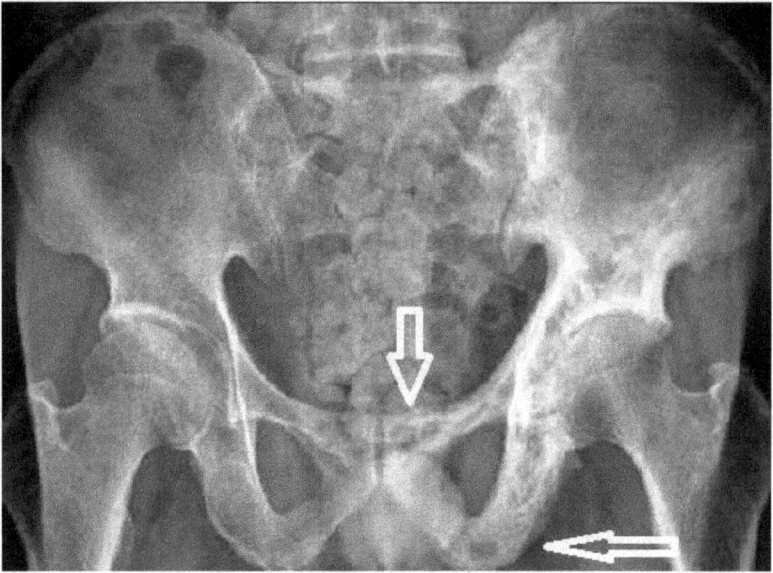

Multiple osteolytic metastasis.[7]

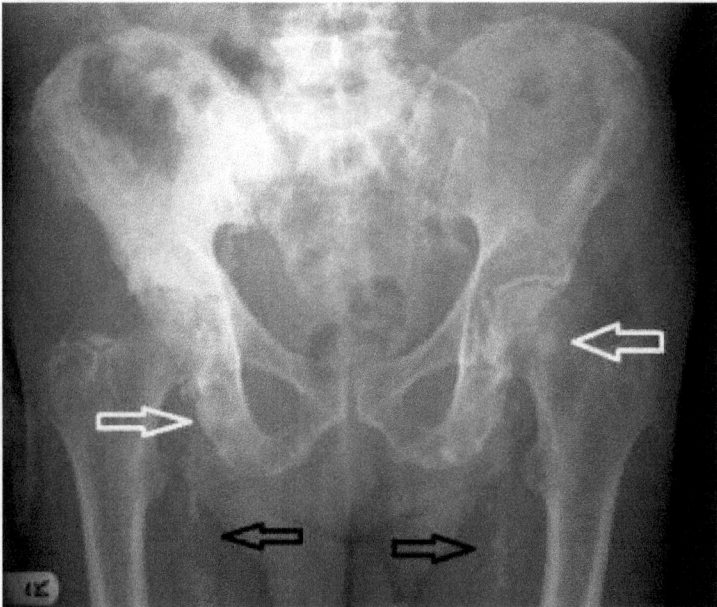

Multiple osteoblastic metastasis from prostate cancer (white arrows). Calcifications of the femoral arteries (black arrows).

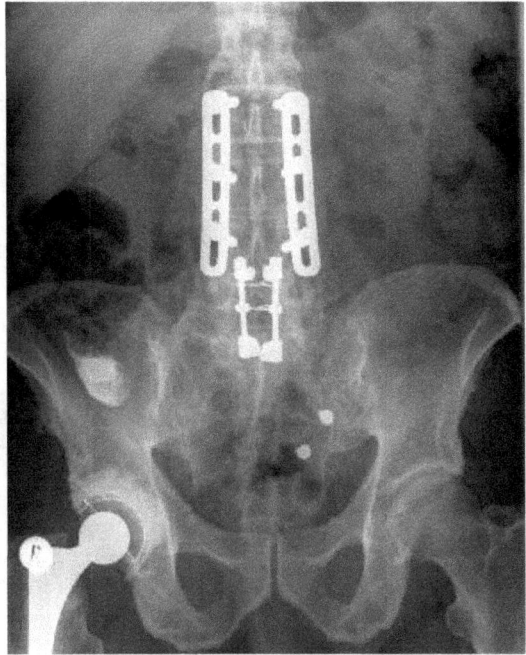

Lumbar spinal fixation.
Right THR and extra-
urinary calcifications.

Spine: scoliosis, degenerative changes like lysis or lysthesis, osteophytes, spinal dysraphism and its level.

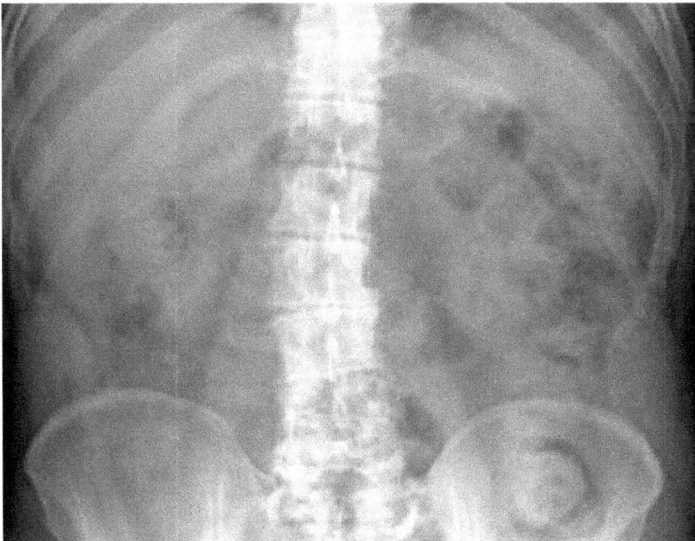

Dextro-convex spinal scoliosis.

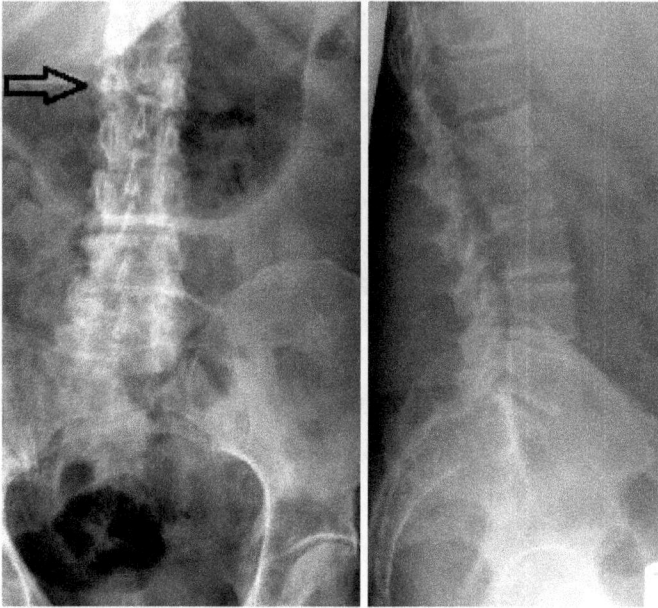

L1 fracture (black arrow), and laeral view.

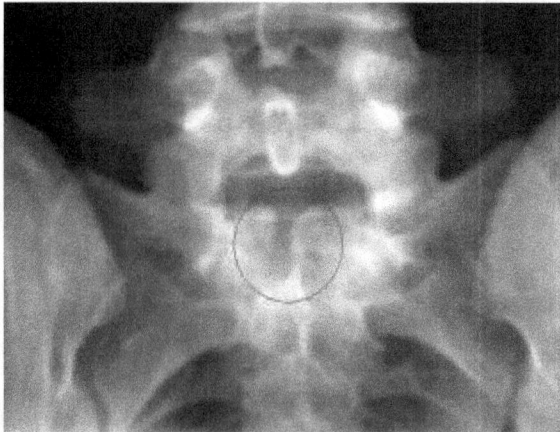

Spinal dysraphism at S1 level (lack of fusion).[8]

Vertebral lack of fusion can present with several urology problems, mainly incontinence and retention. It is associated with spina bifida, myelomeningocoele, tethered spinal cord, tight filum terminale and dermal sinus tracts.

Pelvic girdle: hip replacement, scars of fractures or retro pubic sutures. Paget's disease is a chronic condition and results in enlarged and dysmorphic bones. It is caused by an excessive breakdown and re-formation of bone, followed by disorganized remodelling. The affected bones weaken and become painful. It is frequently confused with osteoblastic bone metastases (like in advanced prostate cancer).

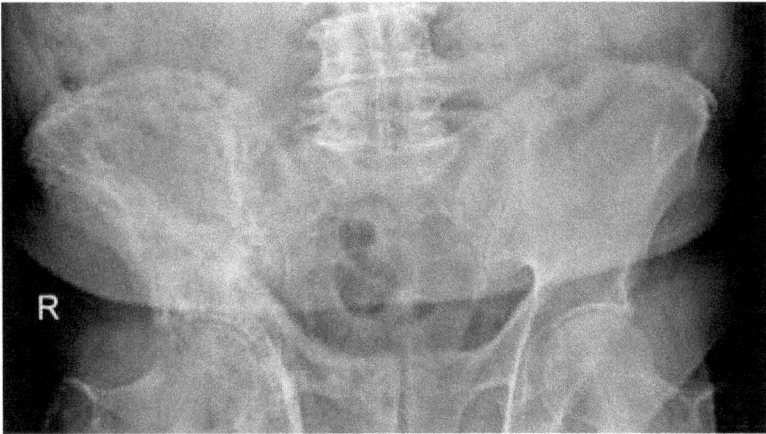

Paget's disease of right iliac bone.[9]

Ribs: resection from flank incisions.
Proximal femurs.

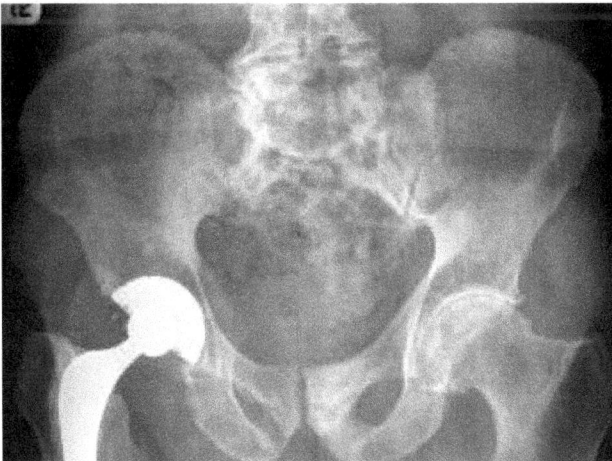

Right THR, osteoporosis and OA of the left hip.

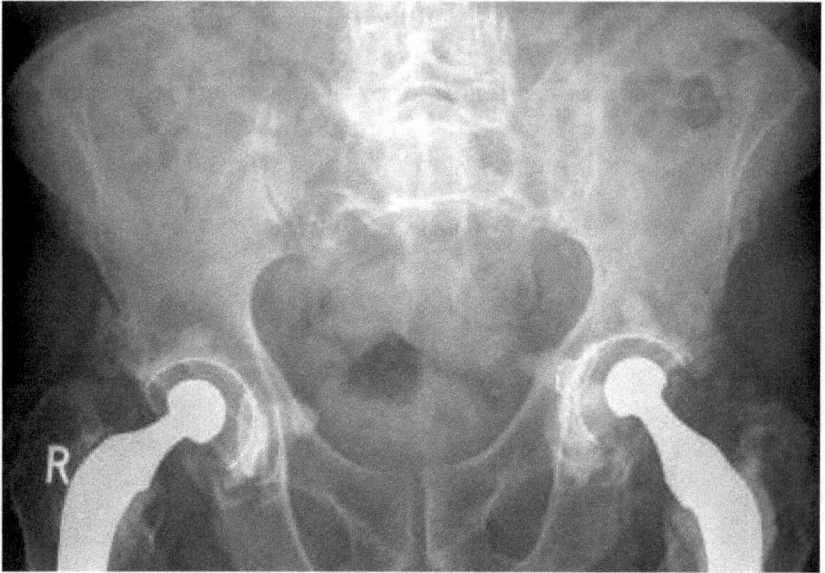

Pelvic bones calcifications related to the bilateral THRs.

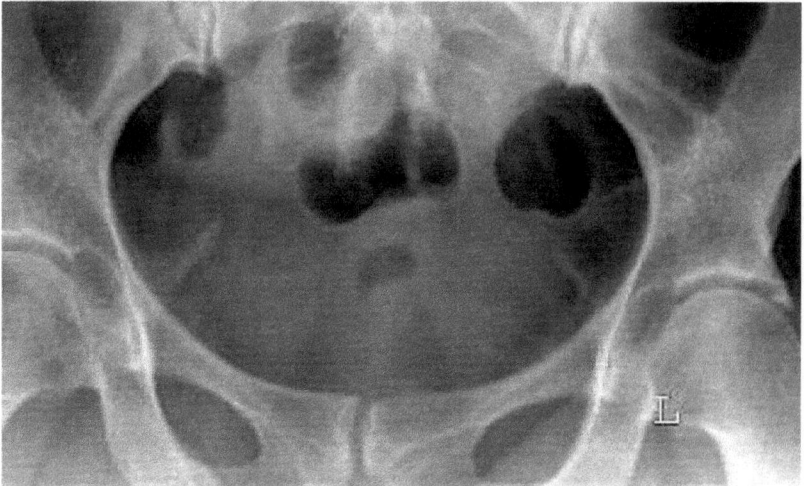

Prominent ischial spines.

b. Muscles.

Psoas shadow: if unseen or substituted by gas it can indicate a retroperitoneal abscess. It is also undefined in retroperitoneal tumours.

c. Subcutaneous tissues.

Gas suggestive of cellulitis (particularly Fournier's gangrene), fat apron.

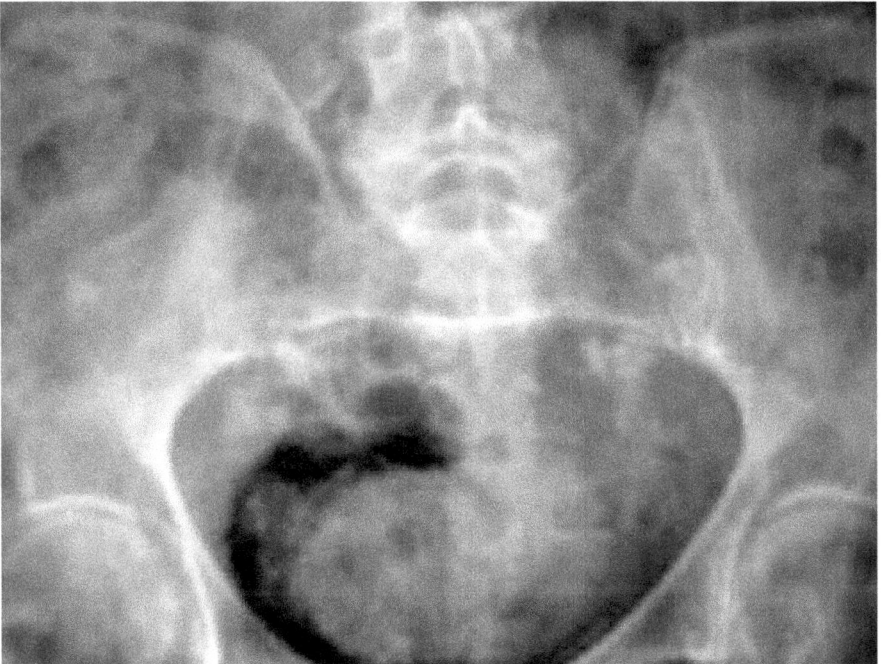

Gas on the right lateral aspect of the bladder shadow in a patient with emphysematous cystitis.[10]

d.   Foreign bodies: piercings, metal fragments, bullets, urostomy and colostomy rings, metal clips, leads and stimulators (pacemakers).

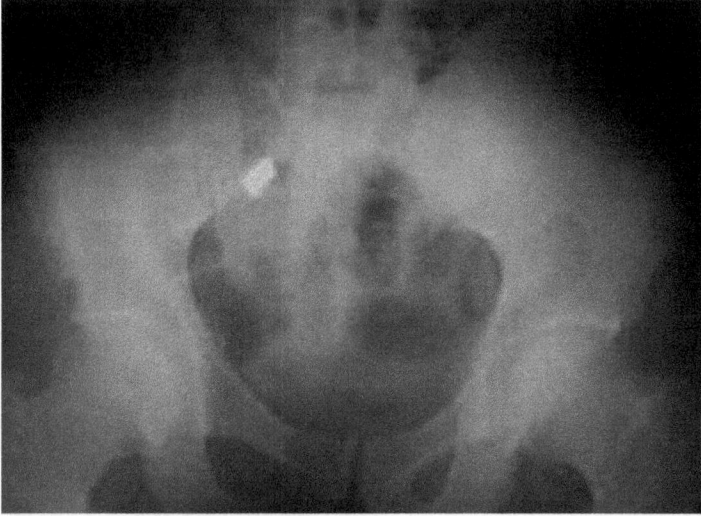

Bullet over right pre-sacral area.[11]

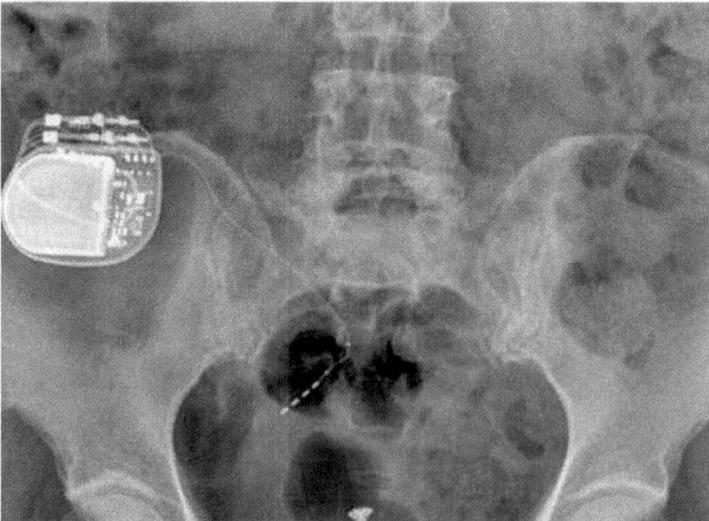

Sacral nerve stimulator (Interstim ®) and lead.[12]

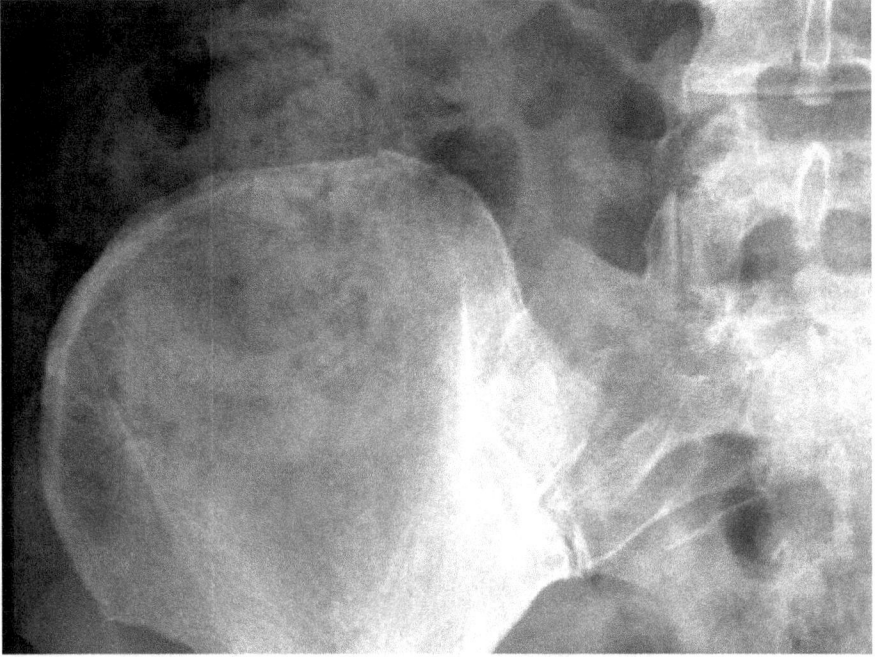

Urostomy ring over RIF.

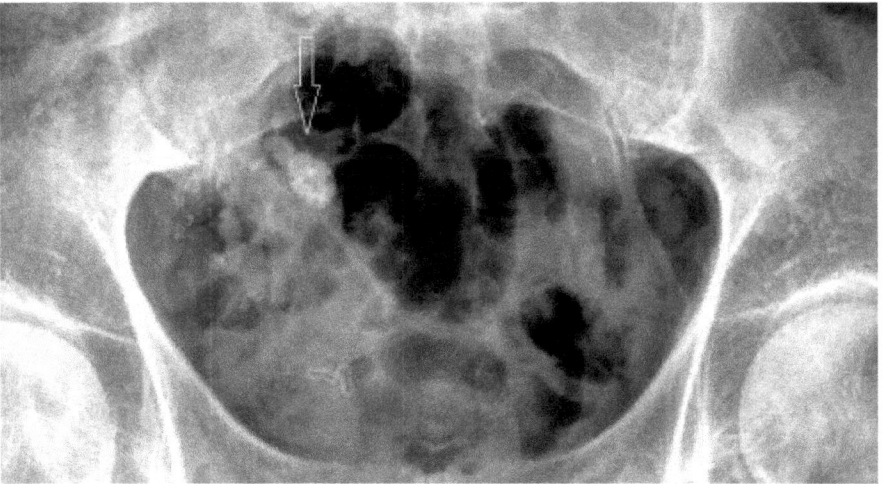

Mesh hernia repair clips (right) and bowel calcifications (arrow).

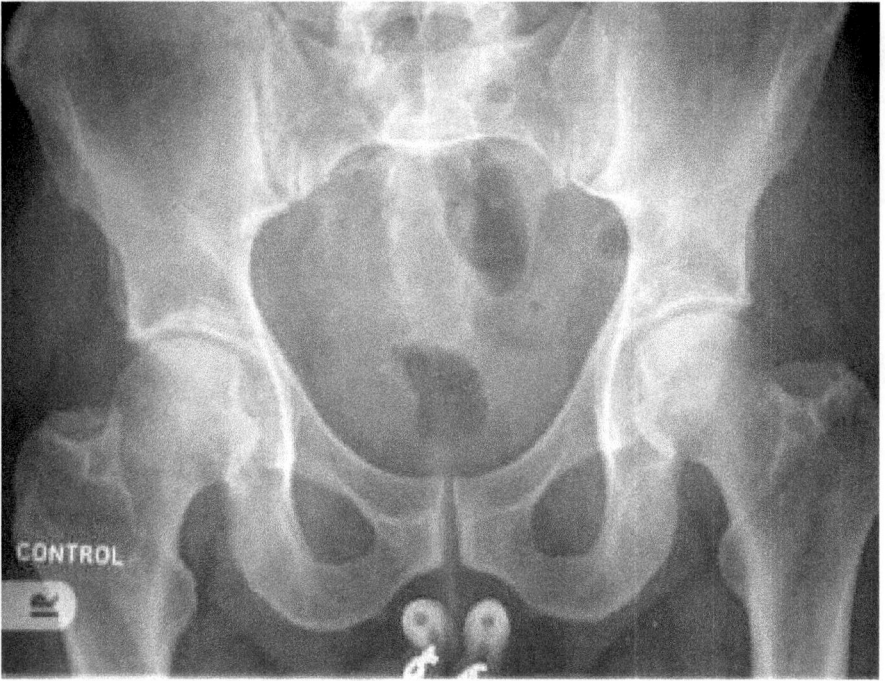

Proximal section of a malleable penile prosthesis under the symphisis pubis.

2. Abdomen and pelvis contents:

a. Kidney shadows.
These are normally located in the lumbar fossae, bean shaped with the mayor axis rotated downwards and outwards (/ \\). As with other organs look for **number** (single unit), **size** (hypertrophy or atrophy), **shape** (especially humps on the external edge suggestive of tumour or chronic pyelonephritis scars), **position** (ptosis, mal-rotation, fusion, pelvic kidney).

The renal pelvis lies lateral to the transverse process of L2-L3.

The right kidney is usually slightly lower than the left kidney.

b. Bowel.
Normal amounts of air and fluid are seen in the intestines. Normal amounts of stool are present in the large intestine. Rule out intestinal occlusion (increased air and fluid levels). Intestinal gas displacement is frequently caused by a tumour mass.

c. Bladder area.
It lies in the pelvis up to the sacrum and down to the upper third of the pubic symphysis. It will vary in size according to bladder volume (residual). It is usually seen as a mild oval shadow of increased density, comparable to soft tissue. A hypertrophic bladder wall makes it more visible.

d. Ureteral area.
From the renal pelvis (L2-3), it follows the transverse processes line to the pelvic brim, then traversing lateral over the common iliac vascular crossing, and finally inwards parallel to the inferior iliac bone line to reach the trigone usually just above the symphysis pubis. The best way to familiarise with this trajectory is to observe it in the excretory phase of an IVU.

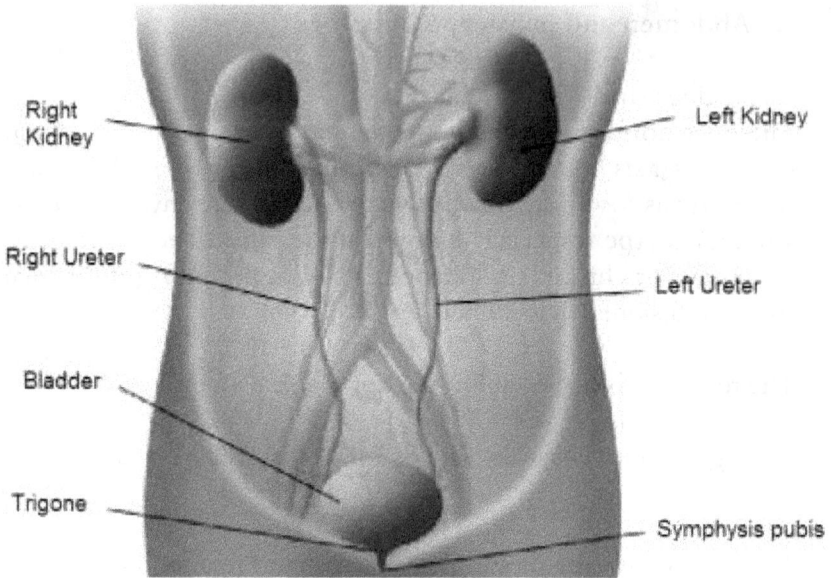

Urinary tract assessed by the KUB.

e.   Abnormal findings.

These can be described by their nature if it is apparent (IUD) or by their density as follows:

- Low density or darker in the film: air or gas as seen in the colon in normal circumstances or in gangrene in the soft tissues or in emphysematous pyelonephritis in the collecting system.

- Medium density or greys in the film: soft tissue, as seen in liver, renal shadows, and full distended bladder. Kidney tumours and lymph node masses have this density.

- High density or whiter in the film: stones, bone or metal and other foreign bodies. The lighter areas in the film normally correspond to bone.

Structures that are dense (such as bone) will appear white, gas will be black, and other structures will be shades of grey.

The four quadrant model.

This is an alternative system to analyse a KUB. Each quadrant contains relatively distinct structures. The four quadrants are defined by two perpendicular lines dividing the abdomen at the umbilicus at right angles to each other. The horizontal line is about the level of L3 and L4 (3rd and 4th lumbar vertebrae). The vertical plane corresponds with the midline, which passes through the xiphoid, umbilicus and the symphysis pubis. The four resulting areas are the right upper quadrant (RUQ), left upper quadrant (LUQ), right lower quadrant (RLQ), and left lower quadrant (LLQ).

Structures found in the **right upper quadrant** include the liver, duodenum, right kidney, right renal pelvis and proximal ureter, hepatic flexure of the colon, portions of ascending and part of the transverse colon.

The **right lower quadrant** contains the appendix, caecum, ascending colon, bladder, right ovary, uterus, right inguinal canal, and right mid and distal ureter.

The **left upper quadrant** contains the left liver lobe, spleen, stomach, left kidney, left renal pelvis and proximal ureter, pancreas, splenic flexure of the colon, and parts of transverse and descending colon.

Within the **left lower quadrant** are the sigmoid colon, descending colon, bladder, uterus, left inguinal canal, and left mid and distal ureter.

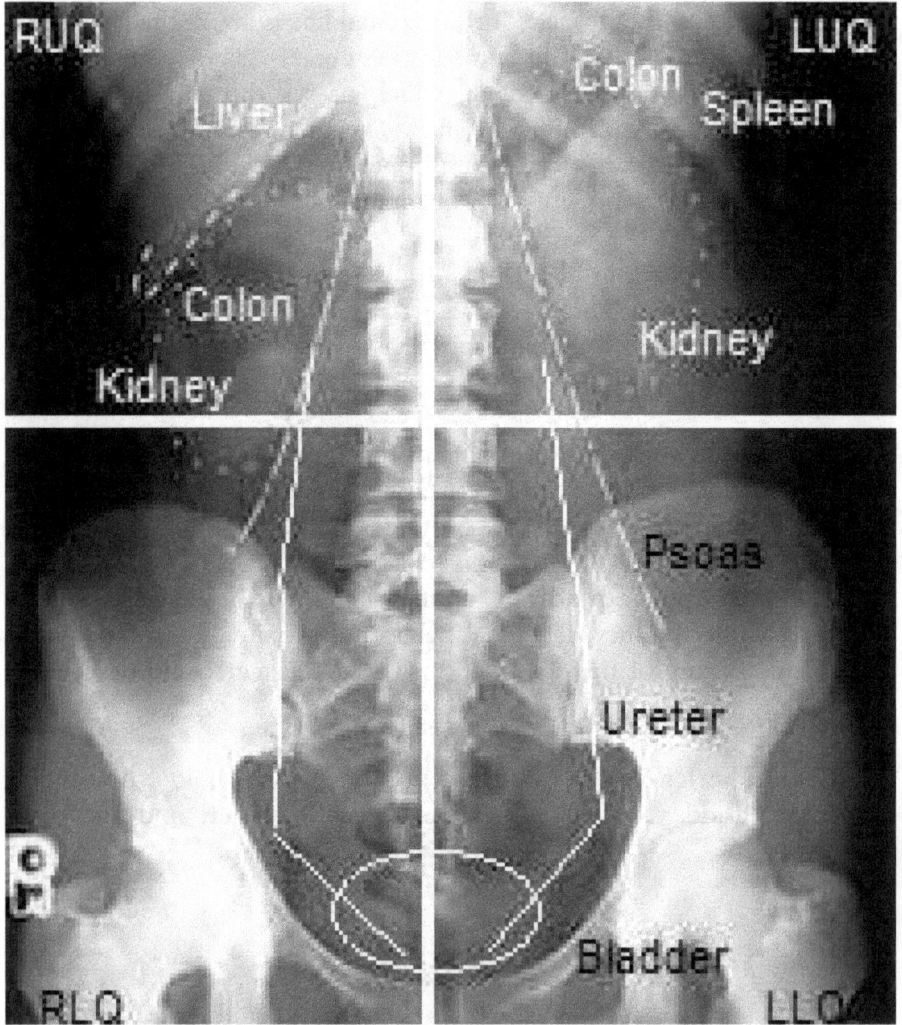

The four quadrant model.

CHAPTER 4. ABNORMAL FINDINGS.

Abnormal findings include:
1. High density or whiter in the film.
2. Medium density or greys in the film.
3. Low density or darker in the film.
4. Mixed density.

1. High density or whiter in the film (calcified images): Urogenital calcifications.

- Urinary stones.

Urinary tract stones (calculi) result from both excessive excretion and precipitation of salts in the urine or lack of inhibiting substances. Men are more commonly affected than women, and the incidence increases with age until age 60. Black race and children are affected less frequently. Renal calculi tend to be recurrent.

The ureter contains 3 areas where calculi commonly become lodged (the pelvic-ureteric junction, the iliac vessels crossing, and the uretero-vesical junction).

A KUB may be sufficient to diagnose lithiasis in patients with known stone disease, otherwise, it is better used combined with an Ultrasound scan (USS)[13] to increase it sensitivity (71%)[14]. At least 80% of urinary stones are calcific, and if clinically significant, they are likely to be seen in a KUB[15]. Non-contrast computed tomography (NCT) sensitivity and specificity (over 95%) is the highest for ureterolithiasis and has become the standard evaluation of renal colic in spite of its considerably higher radiation dose. A reasonable approach is to start with a KUB (sensitivity of 60%[16]), then add an USS to the 40% still undiagnosed (sensitivity increases to 71-78%), and leave the remaining 22-29% of patients to have a NCT. This approach spares at least 2/3rds of the patients of a higher radiation dose, and it is more cost-effective in most centres.

Radiologic classification of urinary stones:[17]

Radiopaque	Poor radiopacity	Radiolucent
Calcium oxalate dihydrate	Magnesium ammonium phosphate	Uric acid
Calcium oxalate monohydrate	Apatite	Ammonium urate
Calcium phosphates	Cystine	Xanthine
		2,8-dihydroxyadenine
		Drug-stones (Section 11.11)

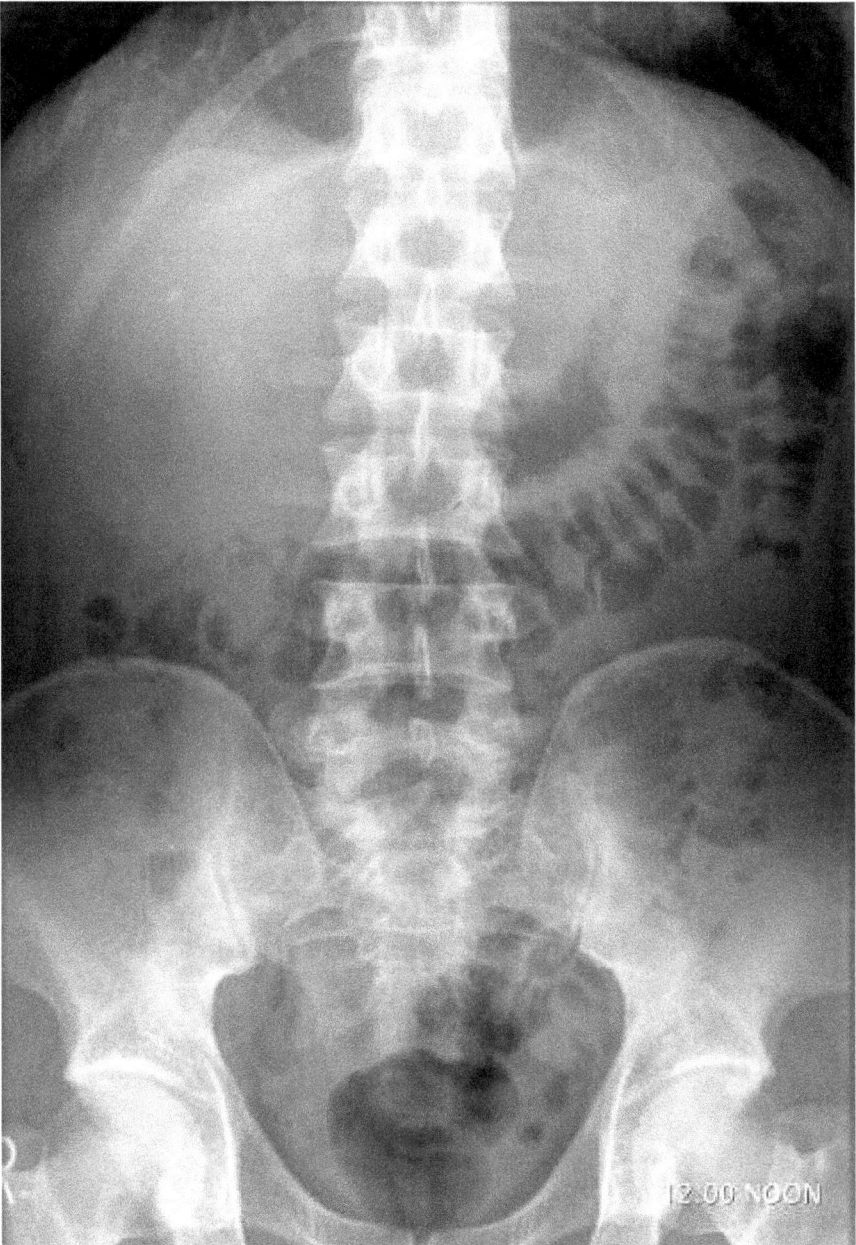

Right kidney stone. Upper calyx (L1-2 level). The right renal shadow
is clearly seen as is most of the colon gas.

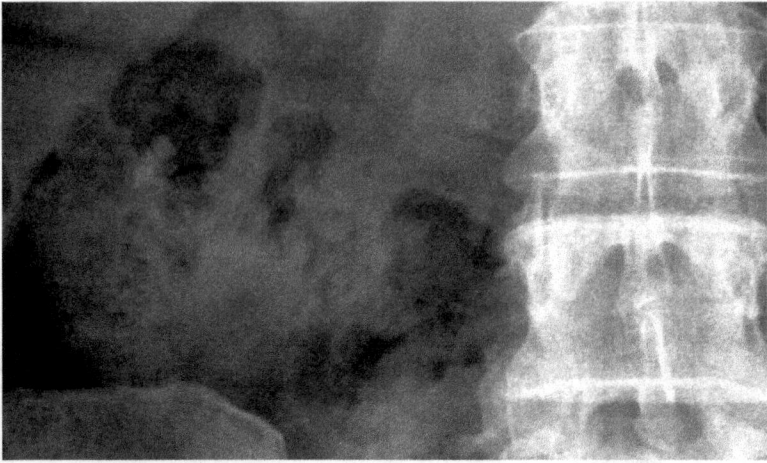

Right kidney stone in lower calyx (L2-3 level).

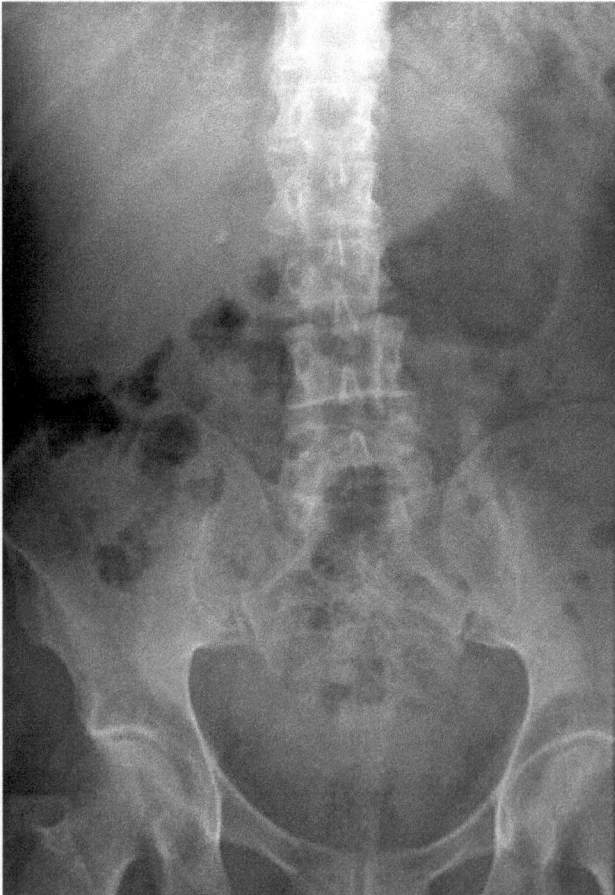

Right kidney stone in a calyceal diverticulum of the upper calyx. Right kidney and liver shadows are clearly seen.

Two radio-opaque renal calculi projected over the lower pole of the left kidney. Psoas shadows seen clearly.

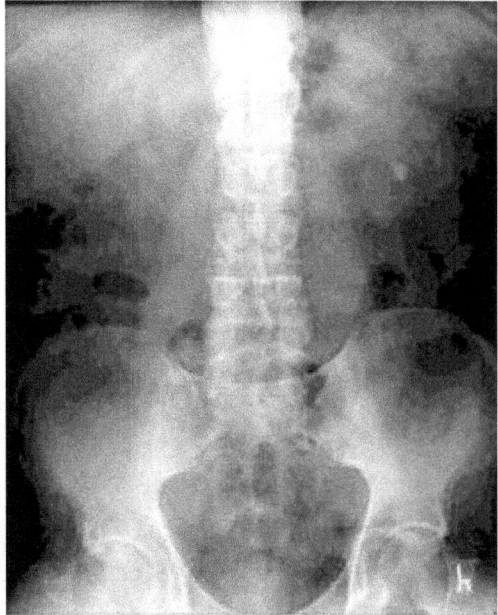

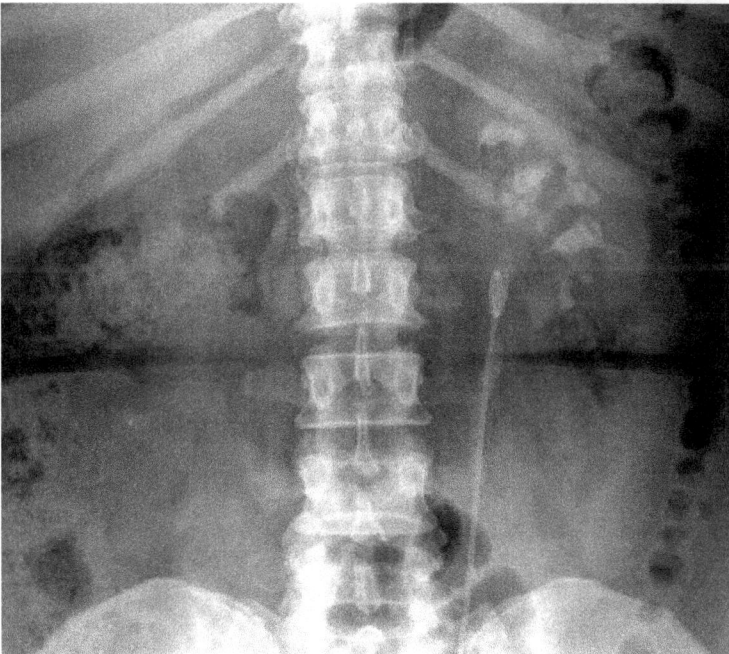

Left coraliform renal stone and JJ stent. Proximal coil (upper) in the renal pelvis at L2 level.

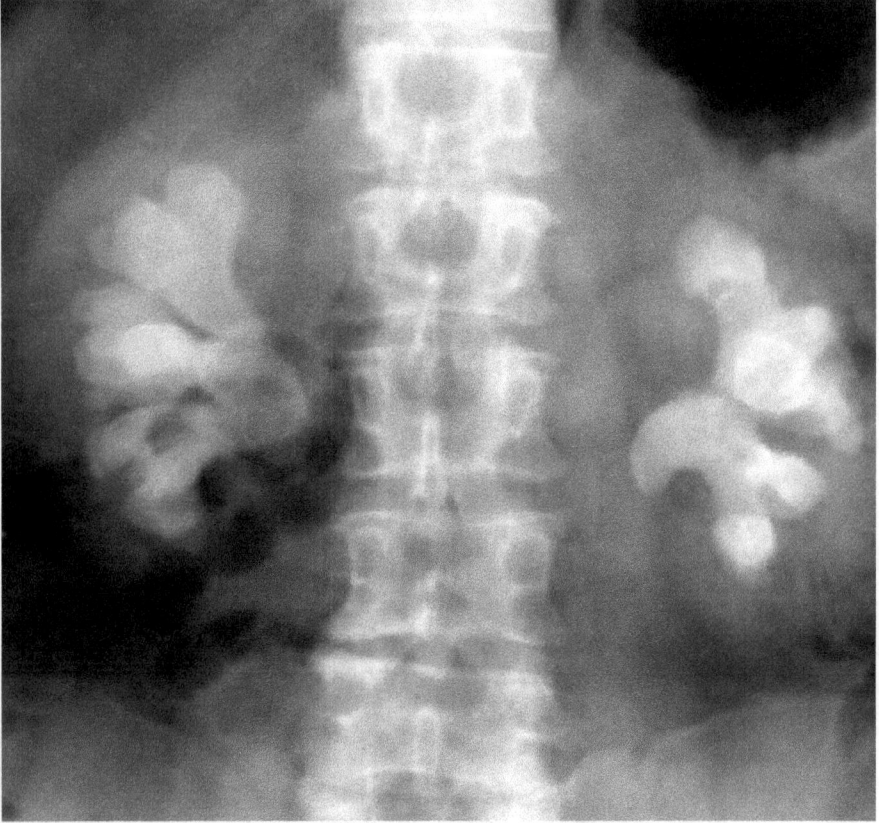

Bilateral staghorn/coraliform stones.

Right renal
pelvis stone
(L2 level).

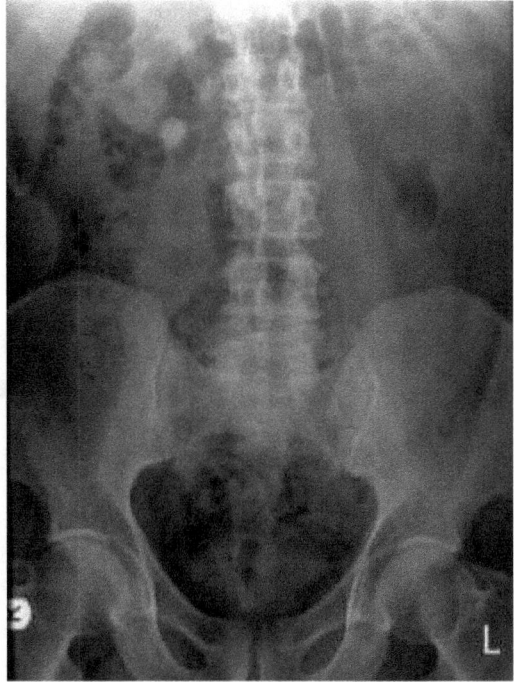

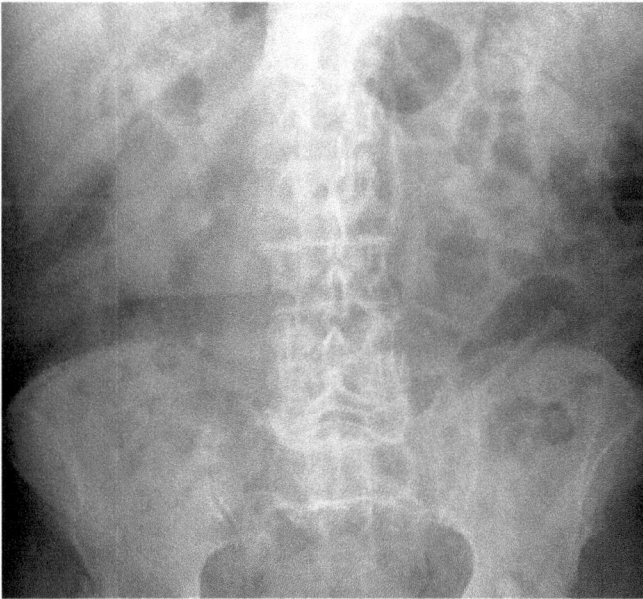

Urinary stones: right renal pelvis (L2-3) and right proximal ureter (tip of transverse process of L4). Right renal shadow is clearly seen.

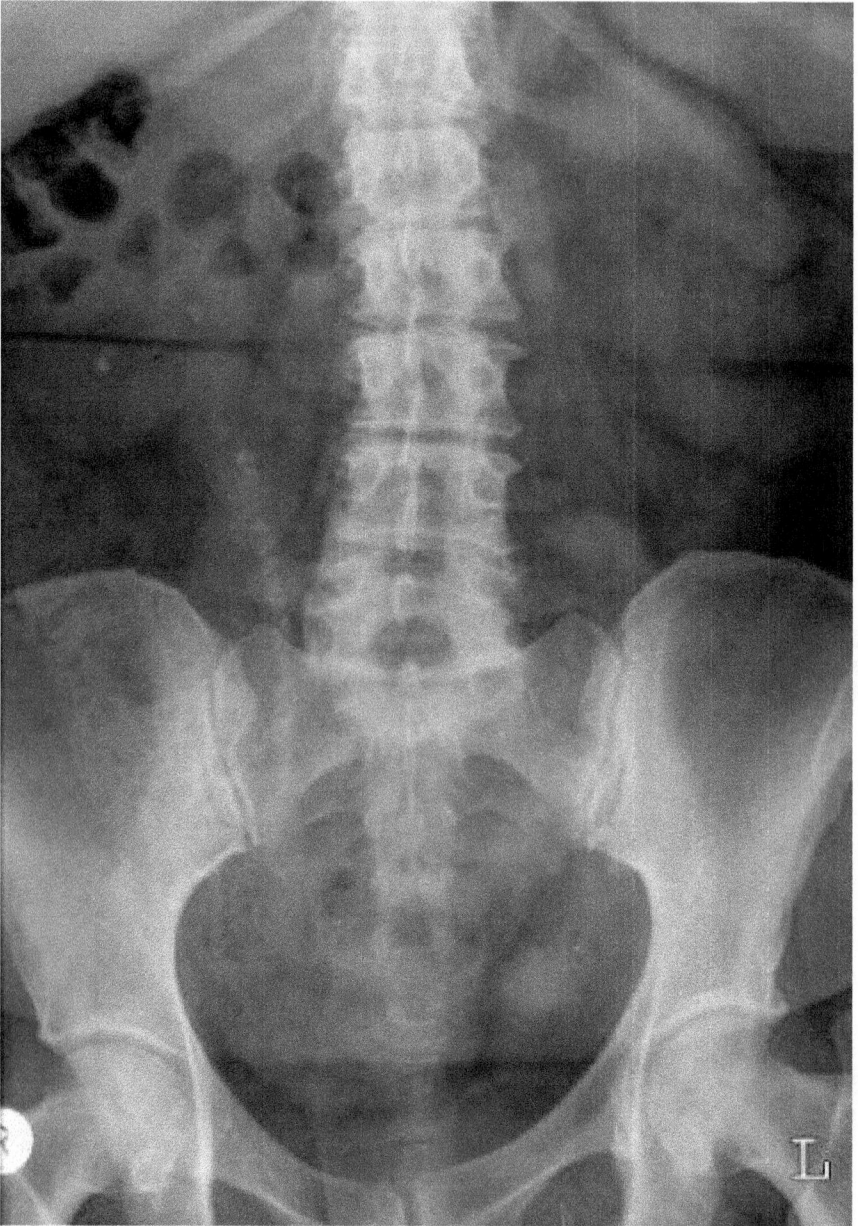

Right proximal ureter Steinstrasse after shock wave lithotripsy of
renal stone. Residual right renal stone fragments.

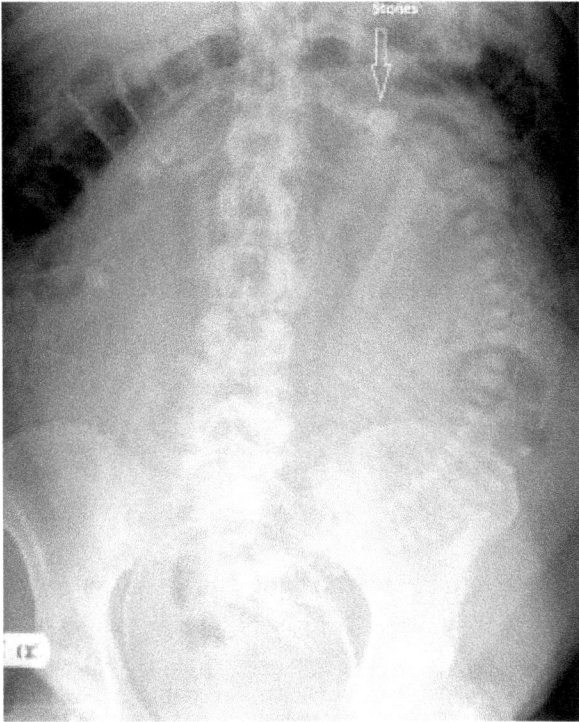

3rd trimester pregnancy with left renal stone.

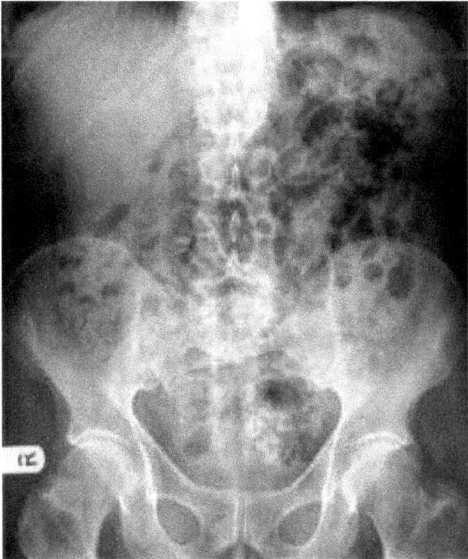

Bladder stone.

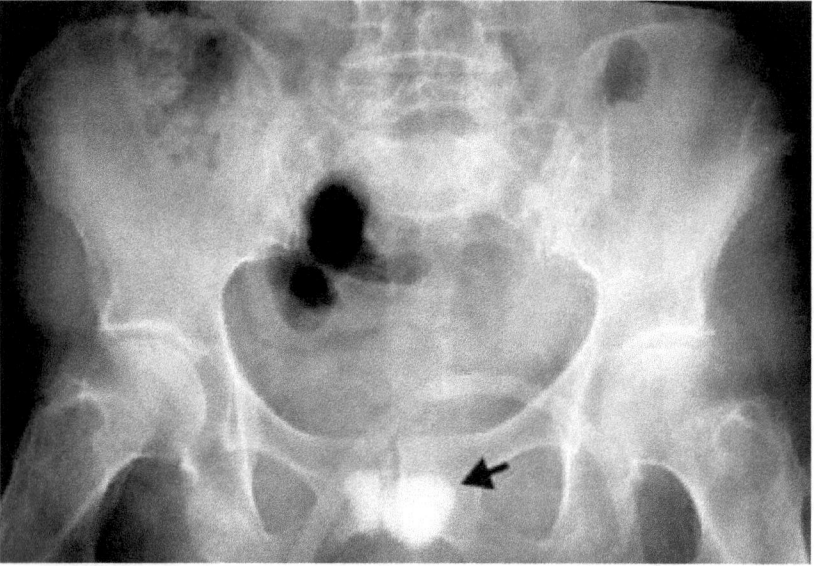

Urethral diverticulum stone (black arrow).[18]

• Hydatid cyst

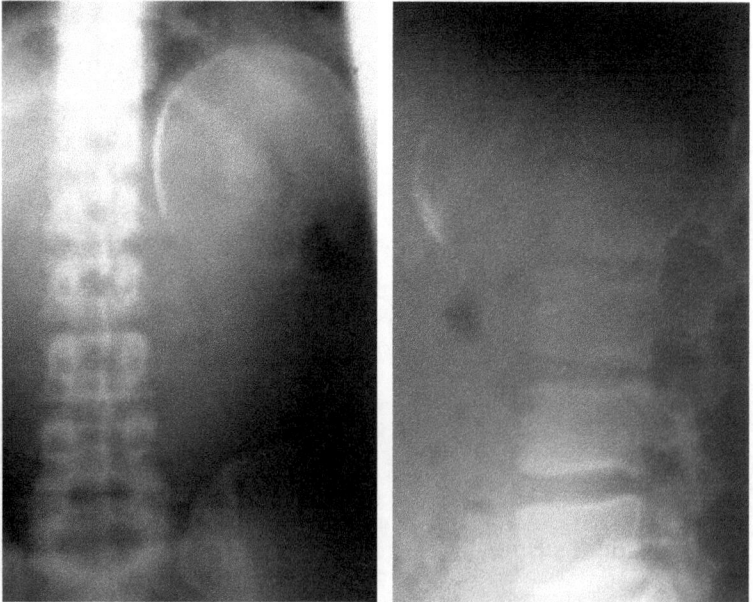

Left kidney hydatic cyst. Lateral view on the left.

- Calcified renal cancer or bladder cancer.

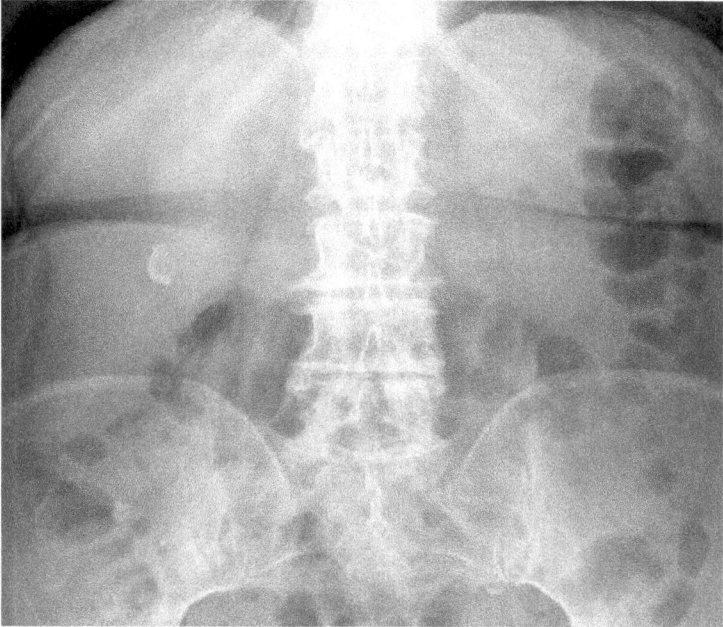

Right renal calcified complex cyst.

- Schistosomiasis

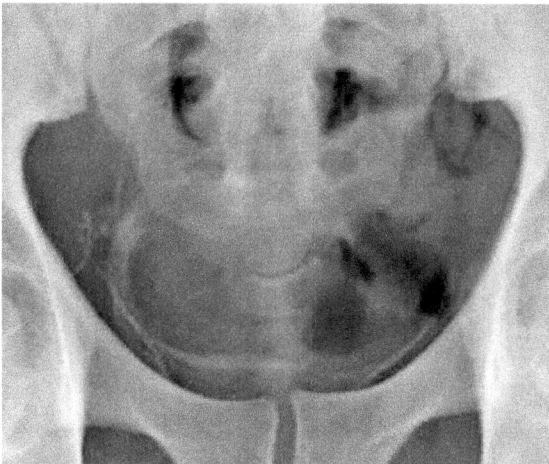

Bladder wall and lymphatic clacifications due to Schistosomiasis.[19]

- Nephrocalcinosis.

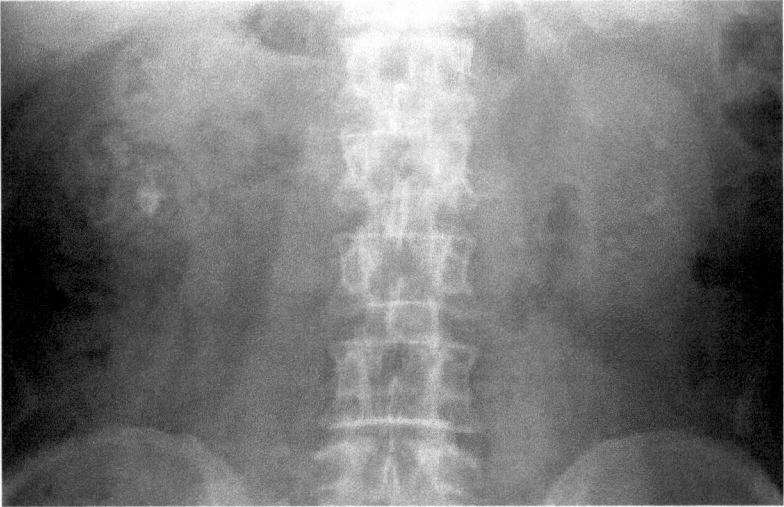

Medullary sponge kidney with nephrocalcinosis.

- Prostate calcifications and stones.

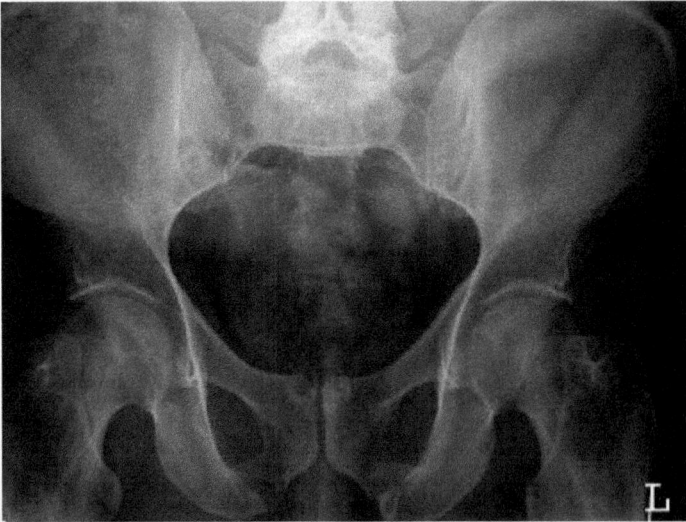

Prostate calcifications seen behind superior part of symphysis pubis.

- Foreign bodies: gastrostomy tubes, NGT, biliary drains, intravascular coils (varicocele treatment) or filters, urethral or suprapubic catheters, drains, Nephrostomy tube, JJ stent, metal clips, surgical materials

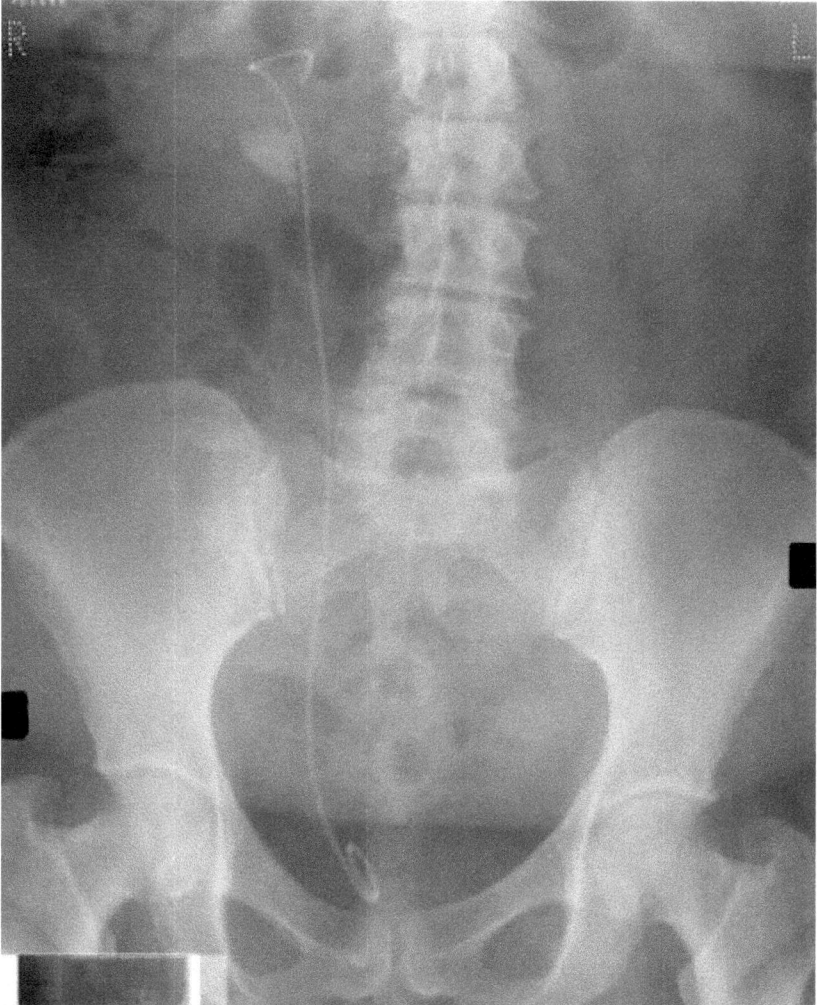

Right JJ stent in place. Right renal pelvis stone (L2 level).

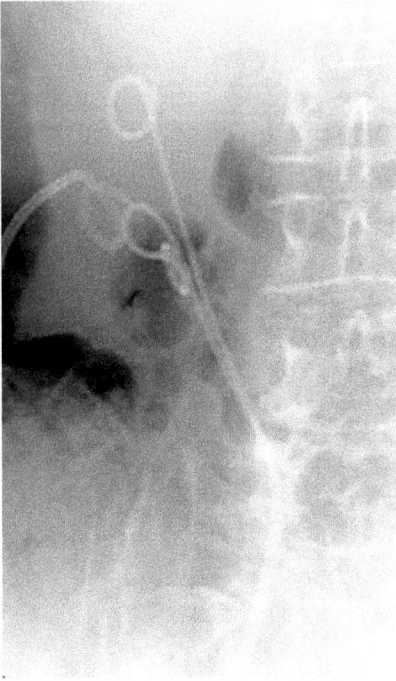

Right Nephrostomy tube and two JJ stents in the right ureter.

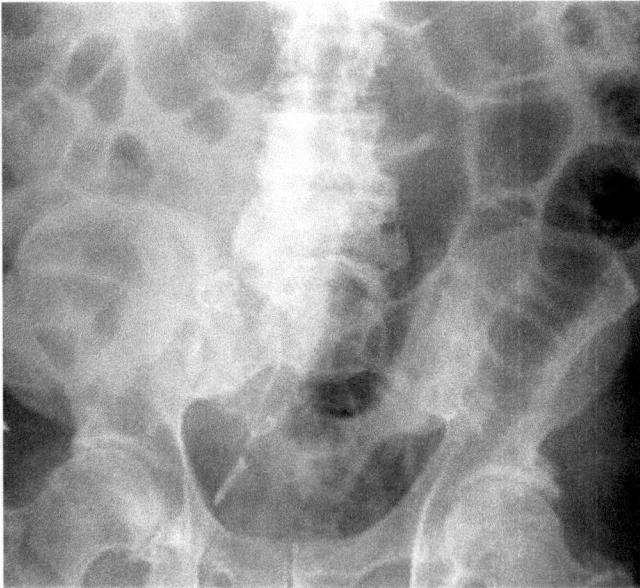

JJ stent in a right pelvic kidney unit.

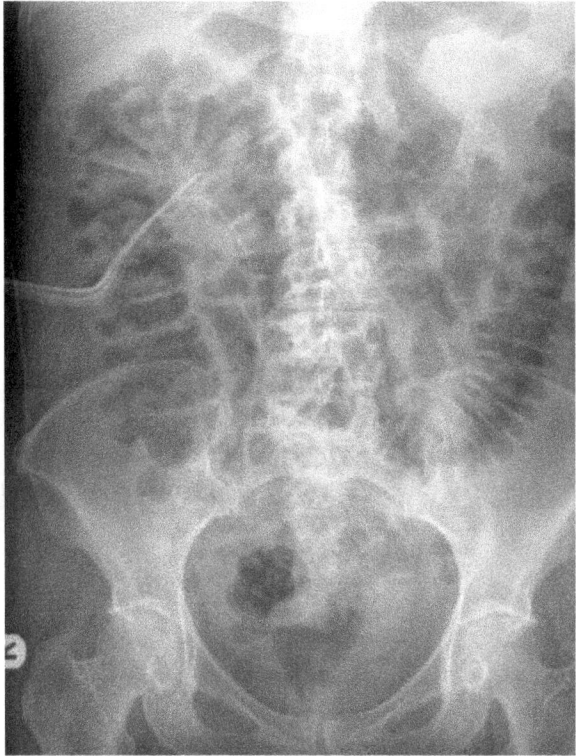

Right nephrostomy tube after PCNL with antegrade ureteral catheter. Gas in the colon without fluid levels (ileus).

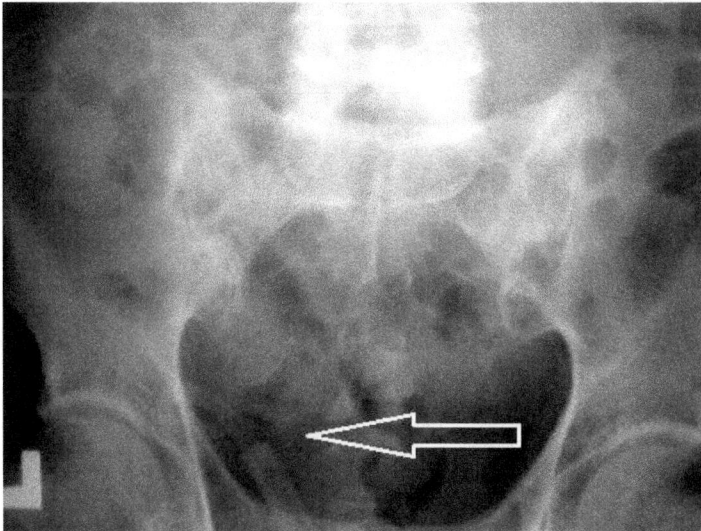

Distal part of urethral catheter over the plevis.

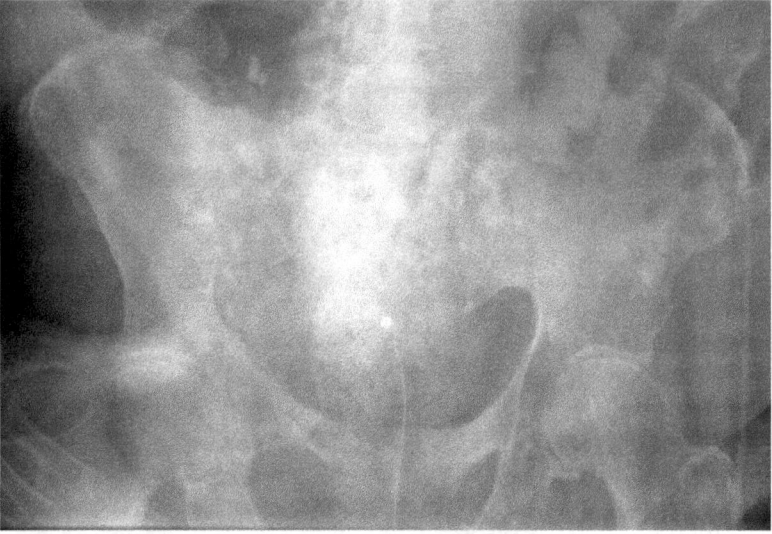

Radio-opaque urethral catheter.

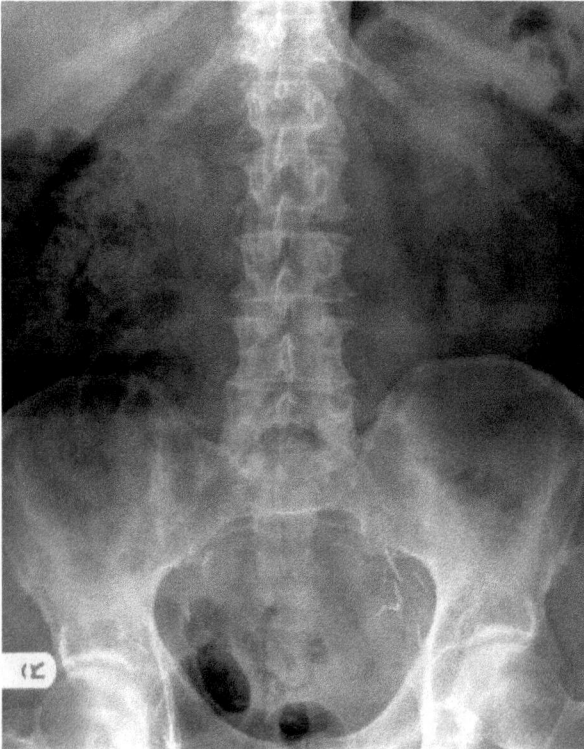

Metal clips from pelvic LND.

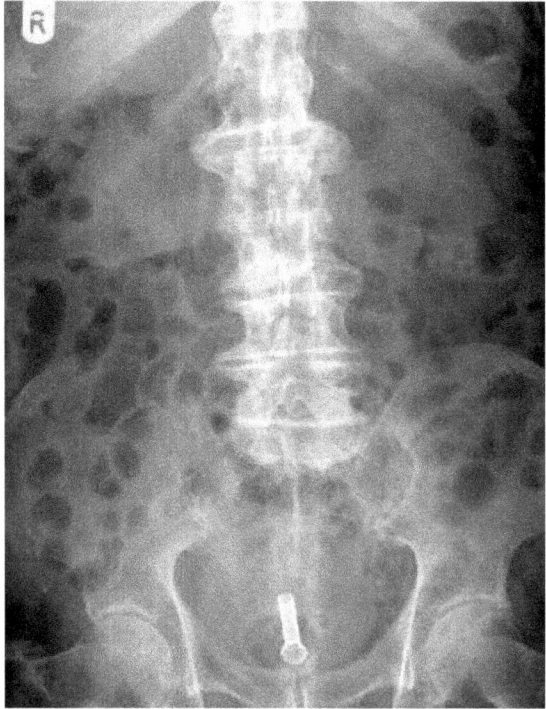

Intra-prostatic metallic stent (Memocath ®). Bladder shadow is clearly seen. Spinal degenerative changes and osteophytes.

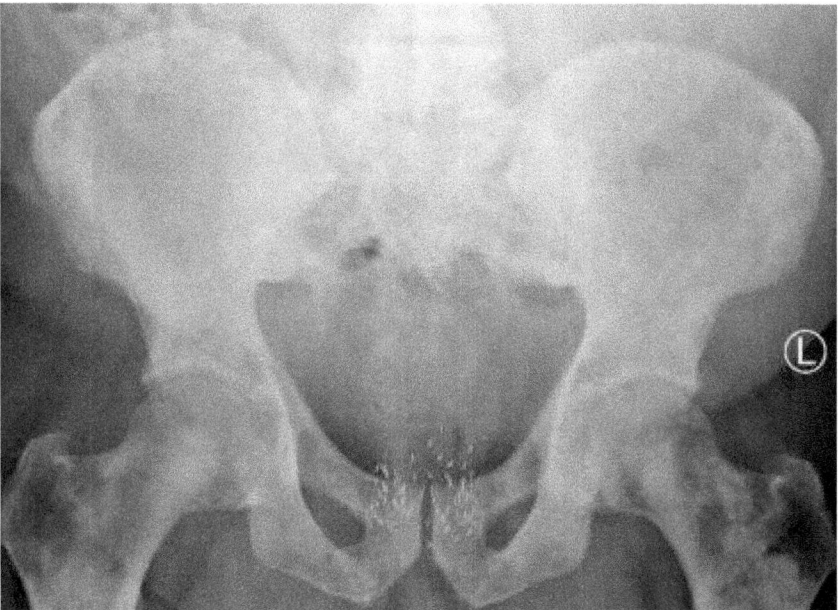

Prostate brachitherapy seeds. Bone metastasis.[20]

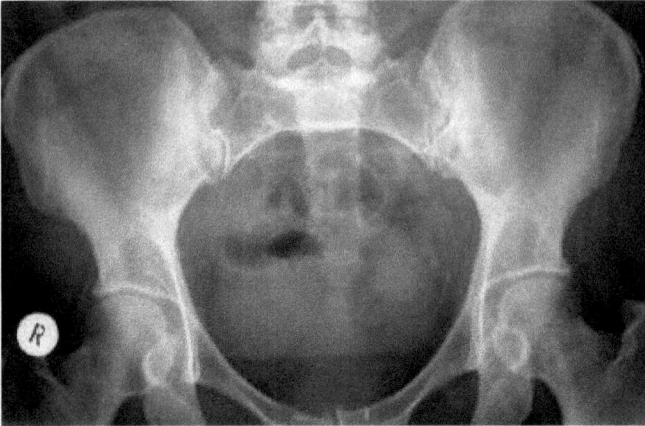

Retropubic calcifications are Stamey bolsters used for para-urethral needle suspension (for correction of stress urinary incontinence).

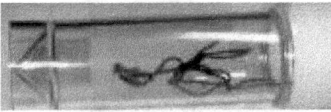

Removed calcified Stamey bolsters.

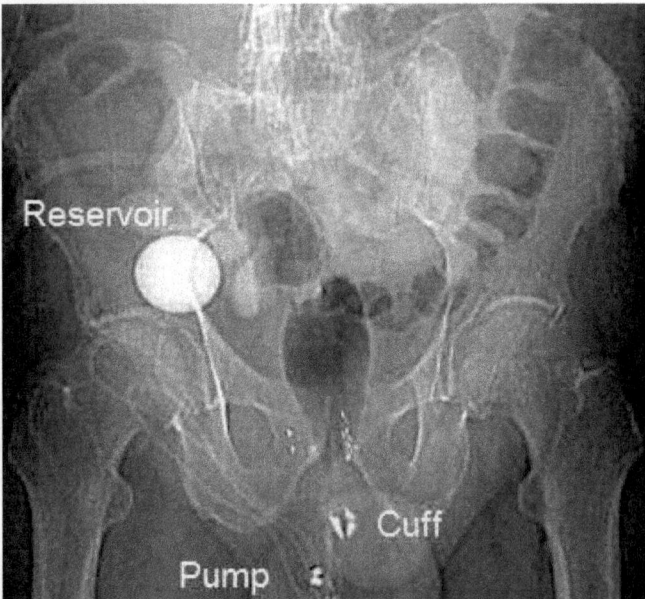

Artificial urinary sphincter. RIF reservoir, right scrotal activation pump, peri-urethral cuff below symphysis.[21]

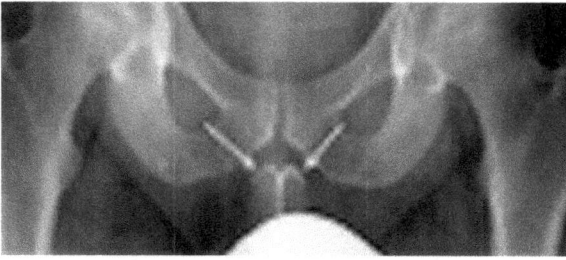

Calcified corpora cavernosa in Peyronie's disease (white arrows). Testes protection shield below.

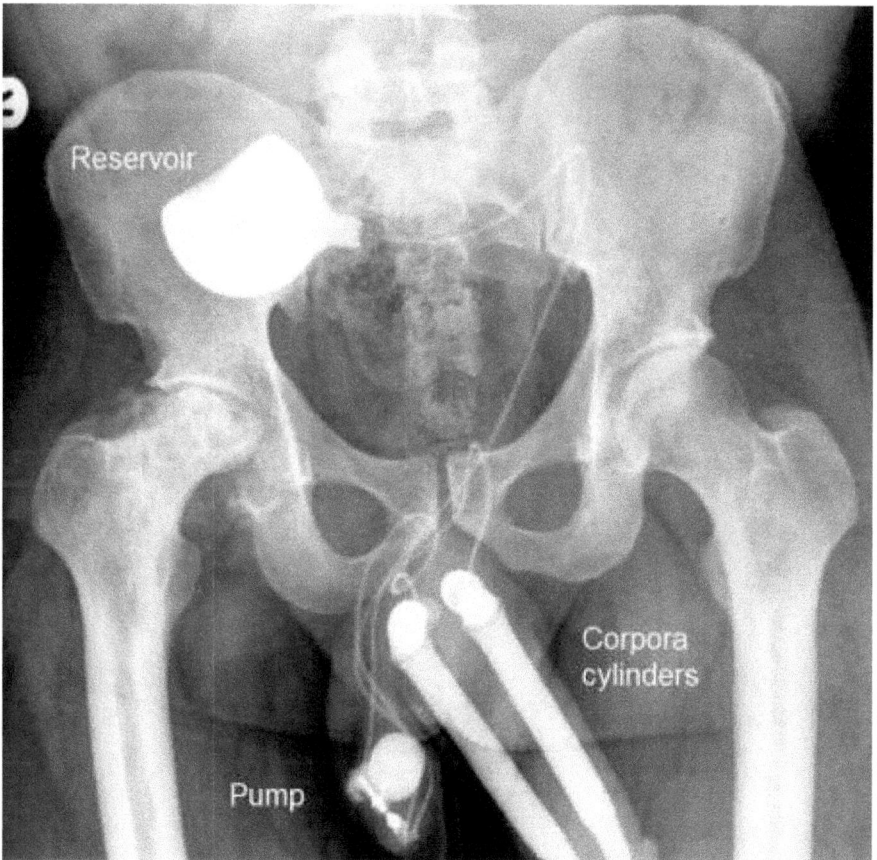

Multicomponent (inflatable) penile prosthesis.[23]

Mr J. Clavijo

Extra-urinary calcifications.

- Porcelain gallbladder.

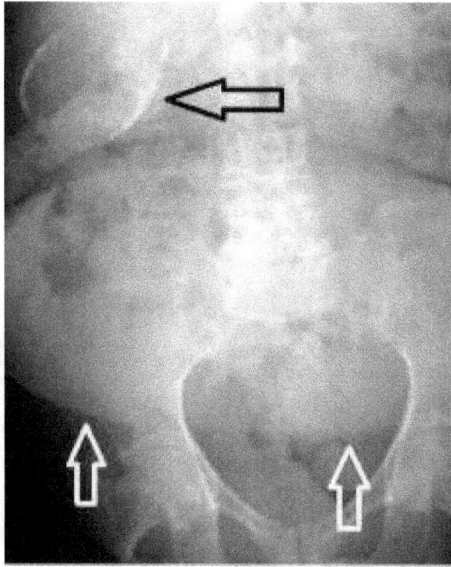

Gallbladder wall calcification (black arrow) and abdominal fat pad apron (white arrows).[24]

- Pancreatic calcifications.

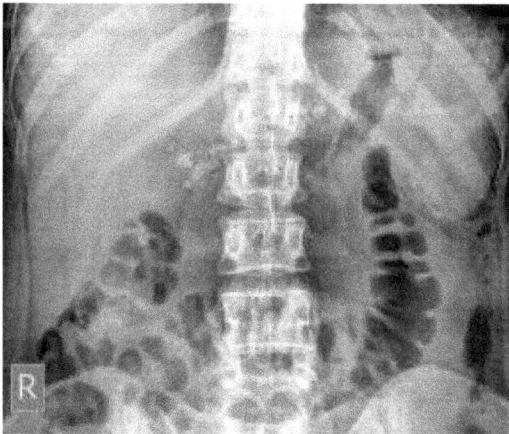

Pancreatic calcifications (white arrows).[25]

45

- Calcified pseudo cyst.
- Calcified abdominal Aortic aneurysm.

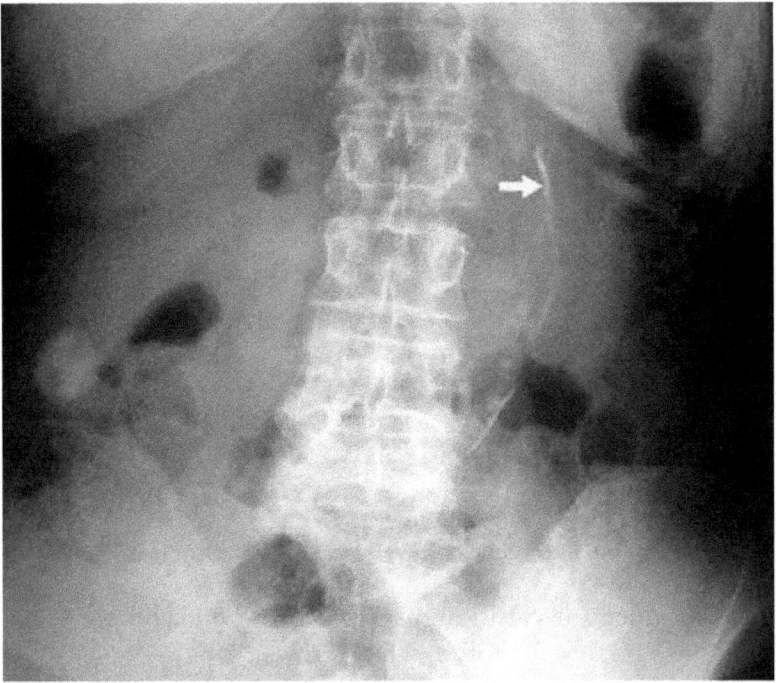

Calcified abdomial aortic aneurism (white arrow).[26]

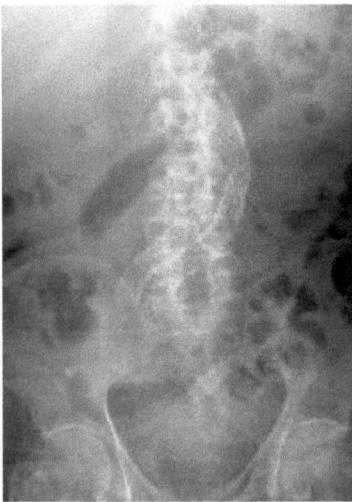

Abdominal aortic and common iliac arteries endoprosthesis.

- Foreign bodies in the intestines.

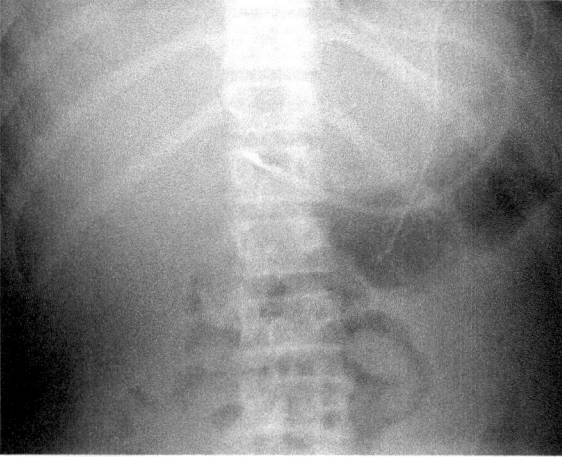

NGT control.

- Vascular calcifications.

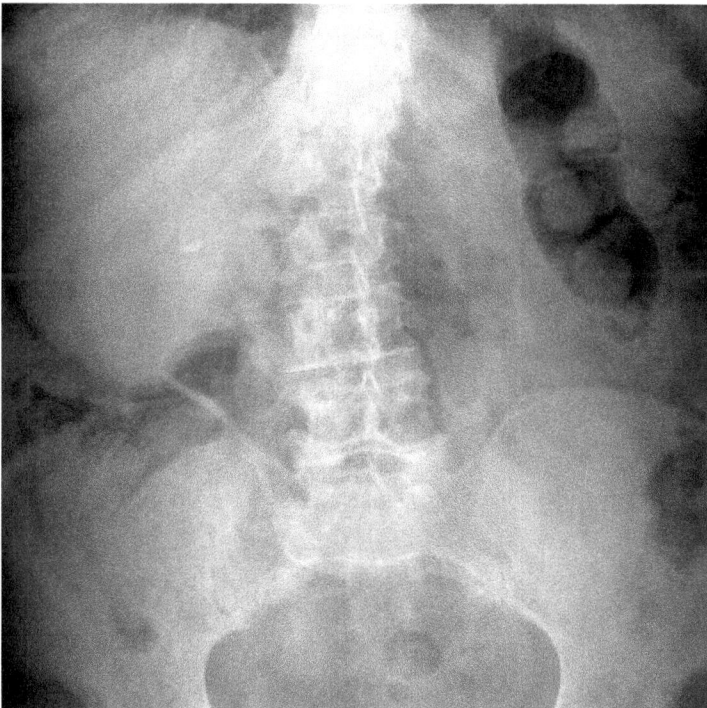

Right renal artery calcification.

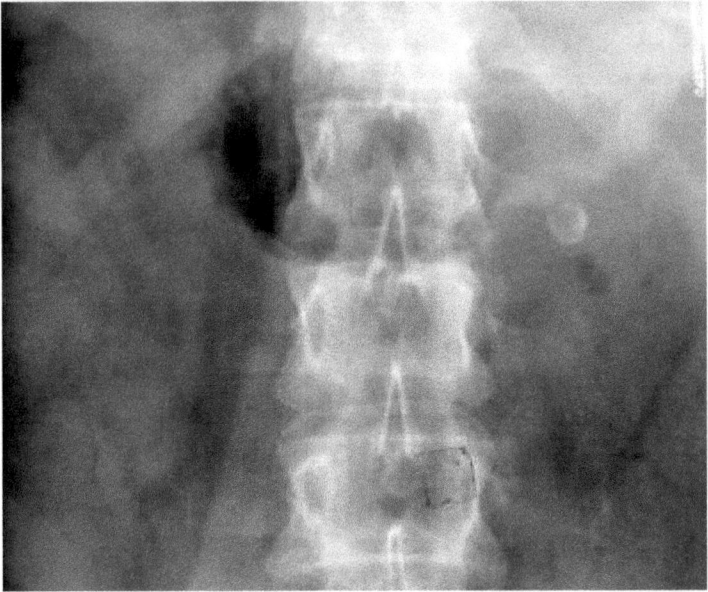

Splenic artery calcified aneurism.[27]

- Biliary stones

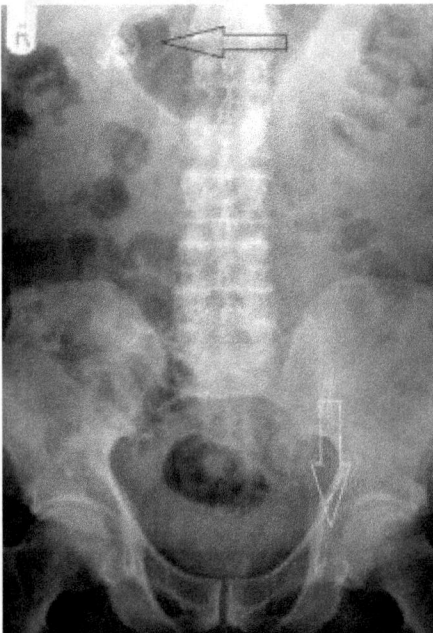

Gallstones (black arrow) and abdominal fat pad apron over the pelvis (white arrow).

Biliary stones
(black arrow).
Right angle of
the colon
displaced
medially (gas).
Fluid density
around
gallbladder.
Pelvic Fallopian
tubes sterilisation
clips.

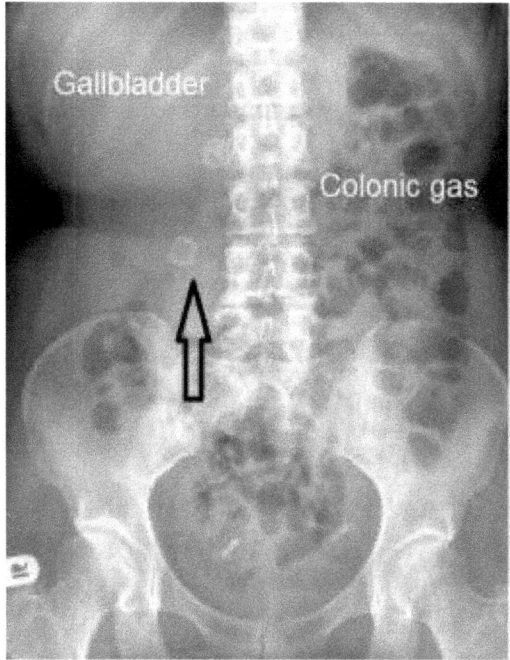

Biliary
endoprosthesis.

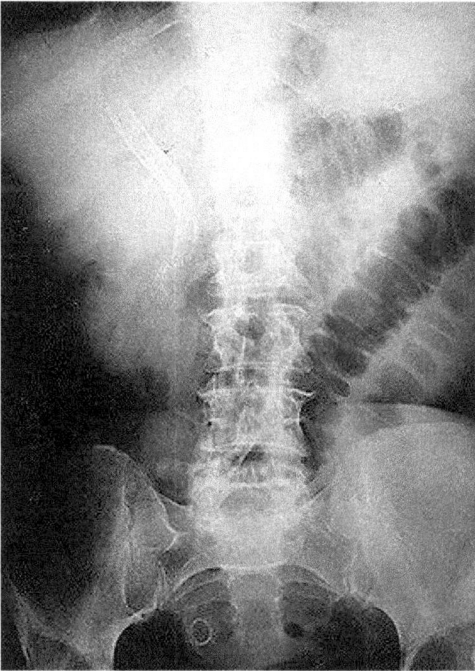

- Phleboliths.
- Calcified lymph nodes.
- Calcific bowel contents.

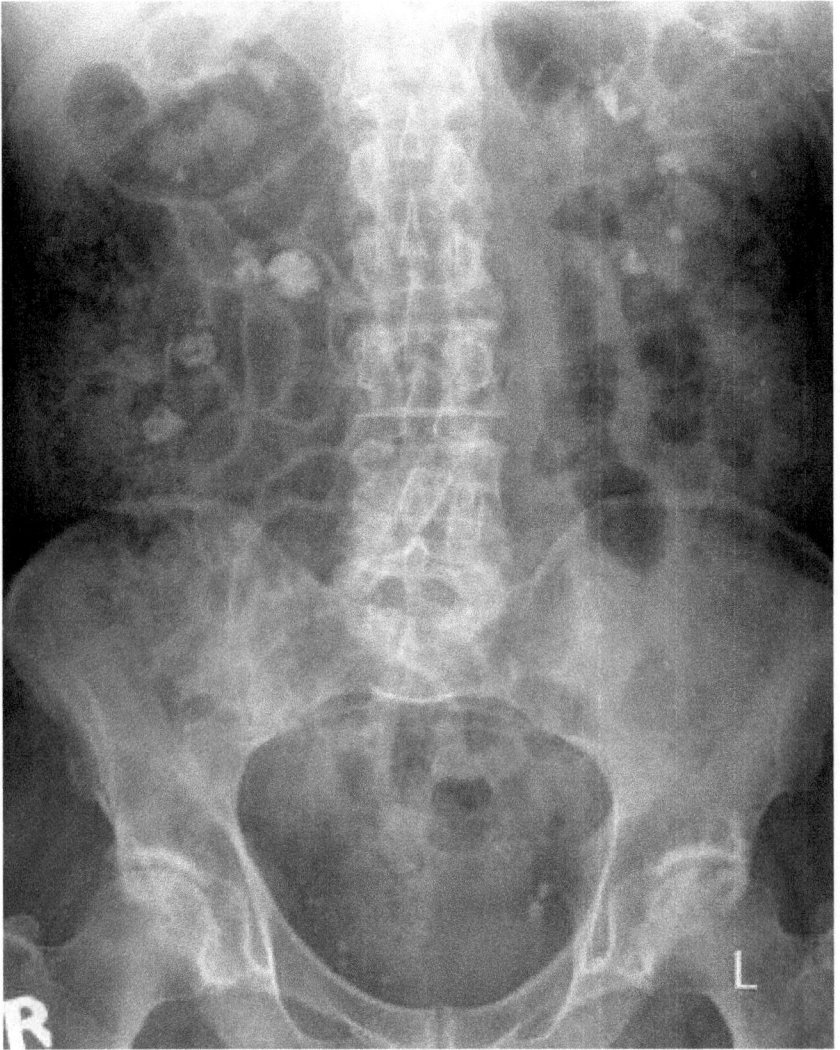

Pelvic calcifications are phleboliths or calcified lymph nodes.
Abdominal calcifications are within the bowel (RUQ) and can be
confused with renal stones (LUQ).

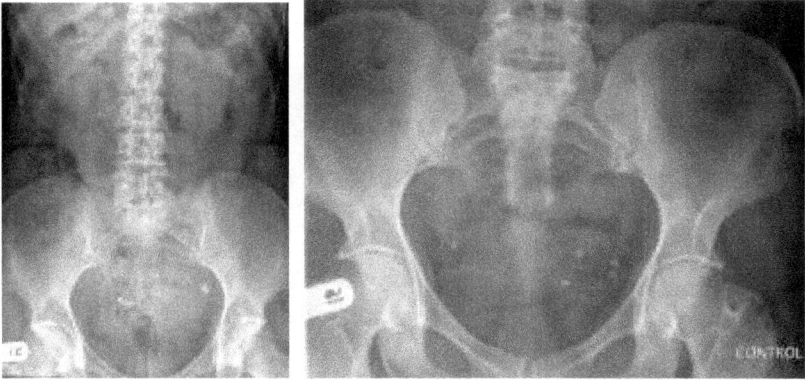

Fallopian tubes clips.

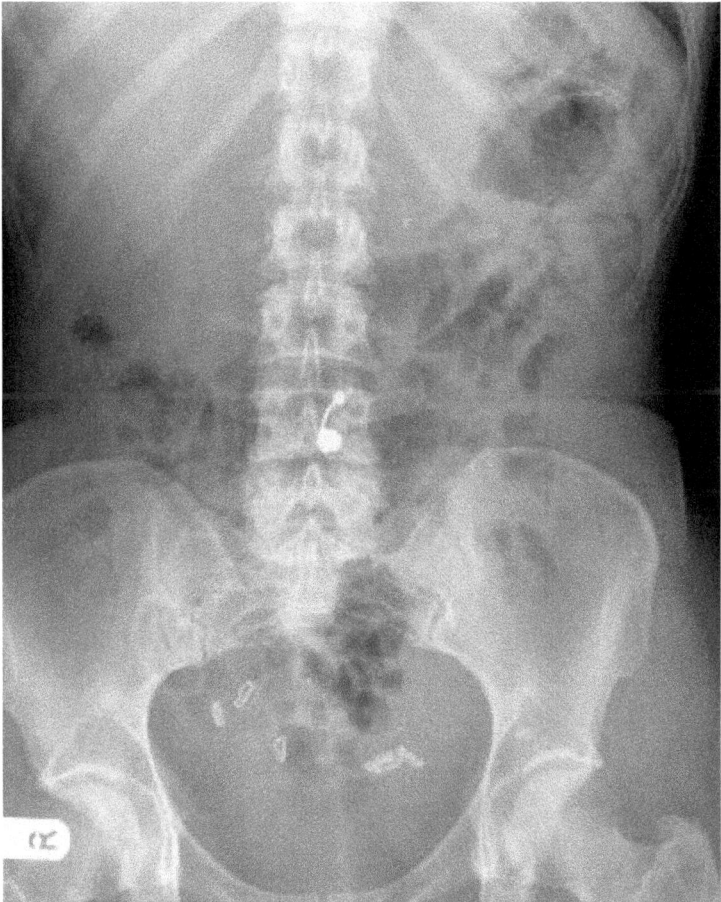

Metallic
abdominal wall
piercing
(umbilical),
gastric stapling
clips and
pelvic
Fallopian
tubes clips.

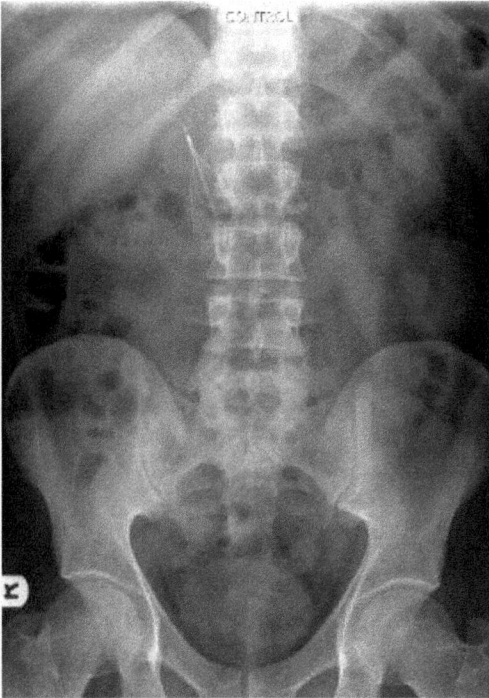

IVC filter to prevent PE in a patient with a left renal tumour. Normal right renal shadow. Full bladder.

- Intra rectal objects

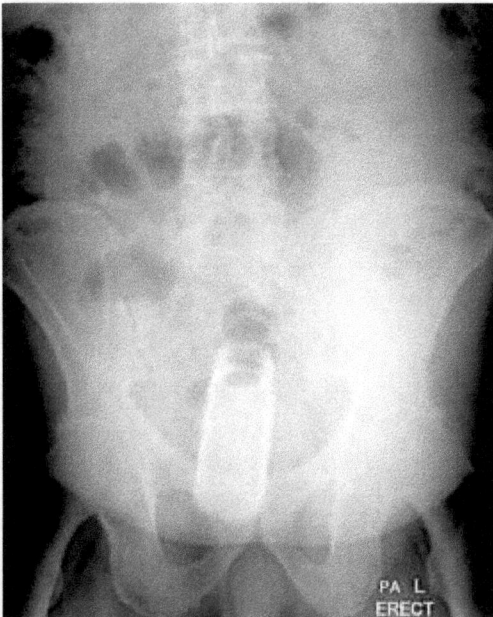

Rectal foreign object was a deodorant bottle.

- Intra vaginal objects.

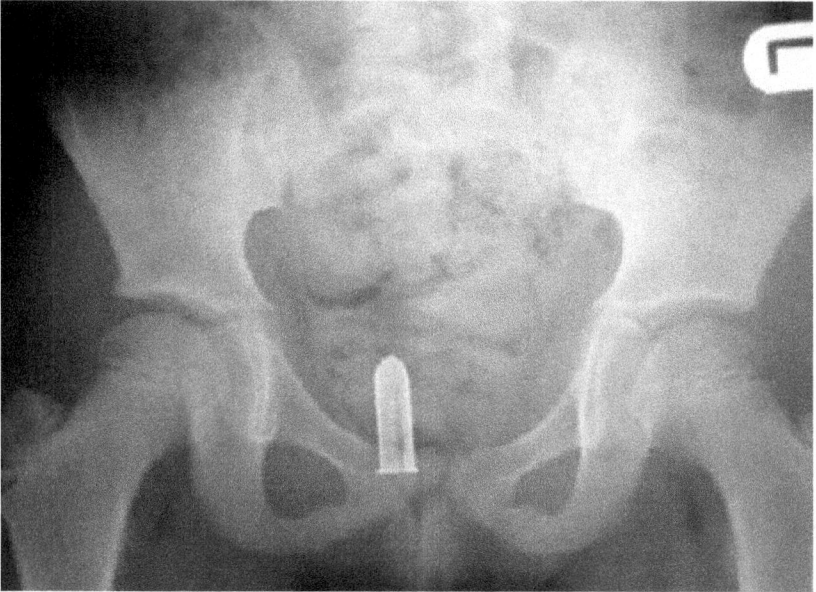

Cap of eyebrow pencil removed from vagina.[29]

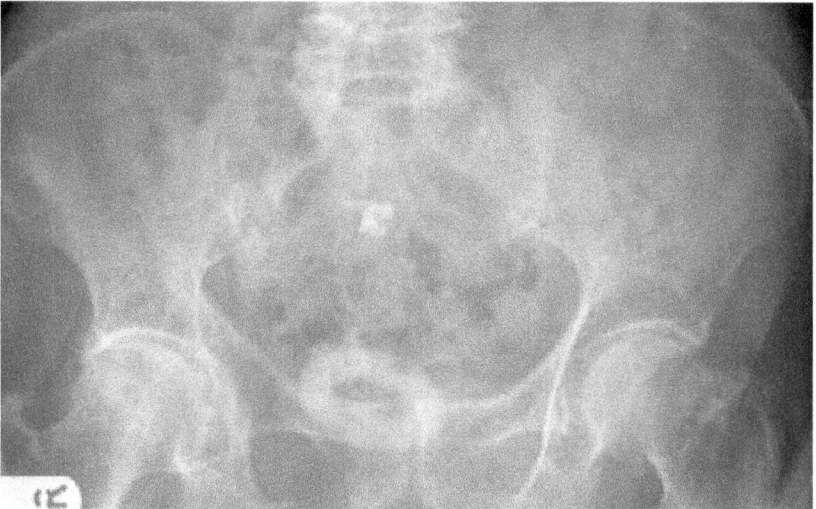

Vaginal pessary. Pelvic extraurinary calcification (bowel/uterine).

- Intra vesical objects

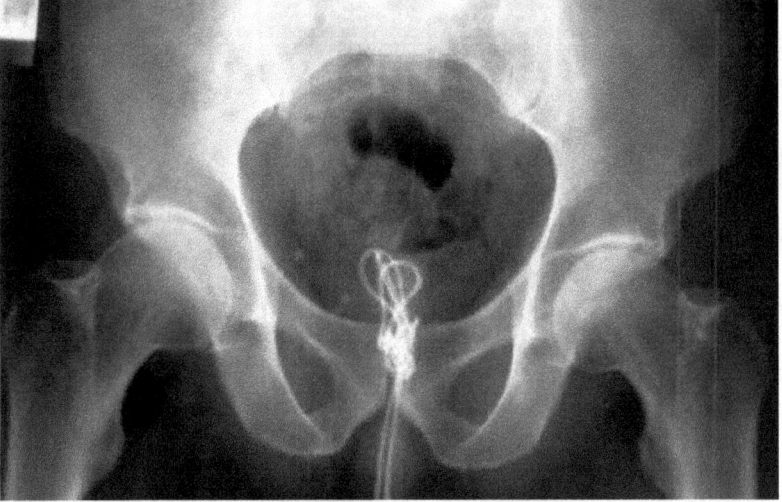

Electrical wire as a foreign body in a male urethra.[30]

- Previous contrast administration, orally, per rectum, intrathecal or I/V and then retained in an obstructive collecting system

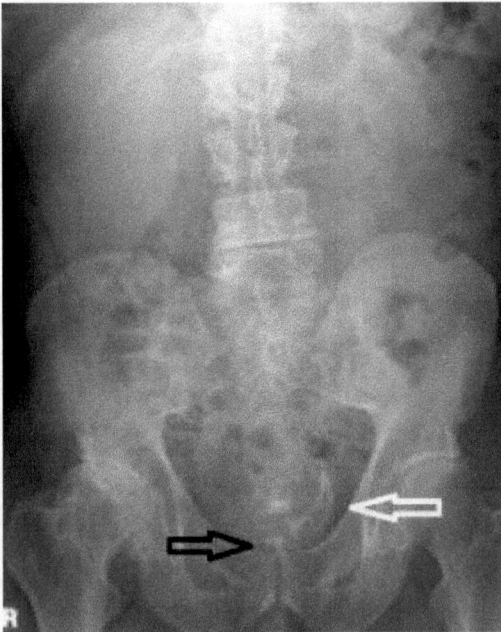

Radio-opaque haemorrhoids cream in the rectum (white arrow) and small bladder stone (black arrow).

- IUD.

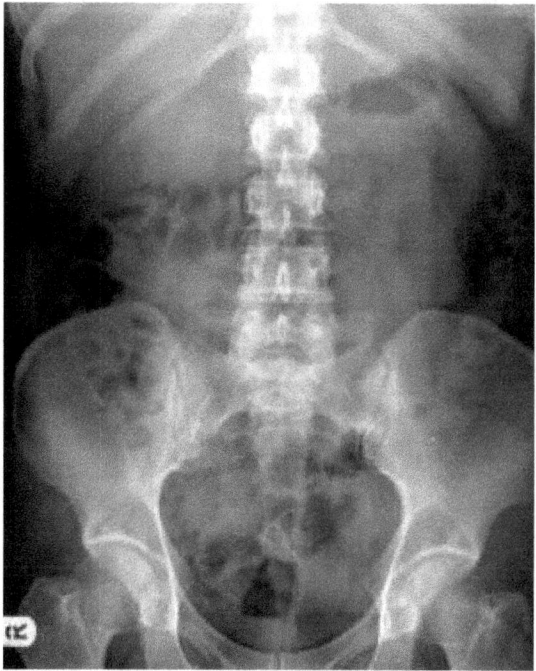

Metallic IUD.
Very clear gas in
the colon.

- Uterine fibroid, calcified.

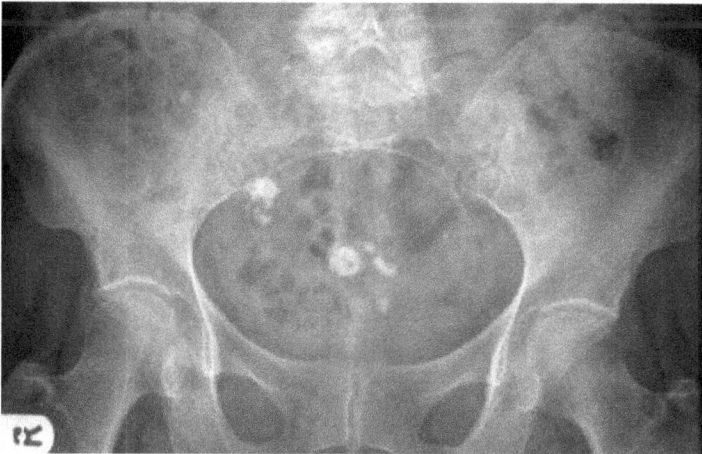

Uterine calcifications.

- Dermoid cyst (benign ovarian teratoma), calcified.

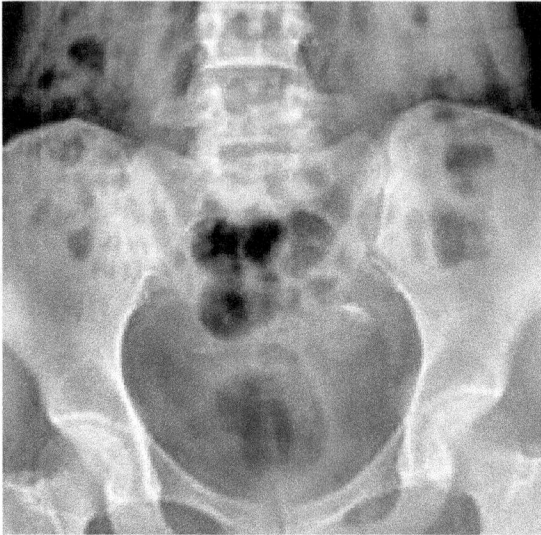

Left pelvic
calcification
resulted in a
dermoid cyst.

- Adrenal calcifications.

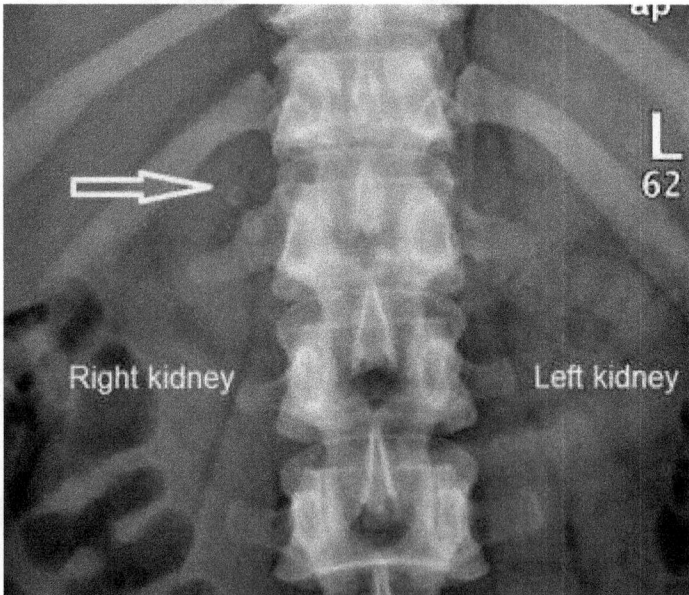

Calcifications of the right adrenal (white arrow). Contour of both kidneys clearly seen.[31]

- Subcutaneous and gluteal calcifications.

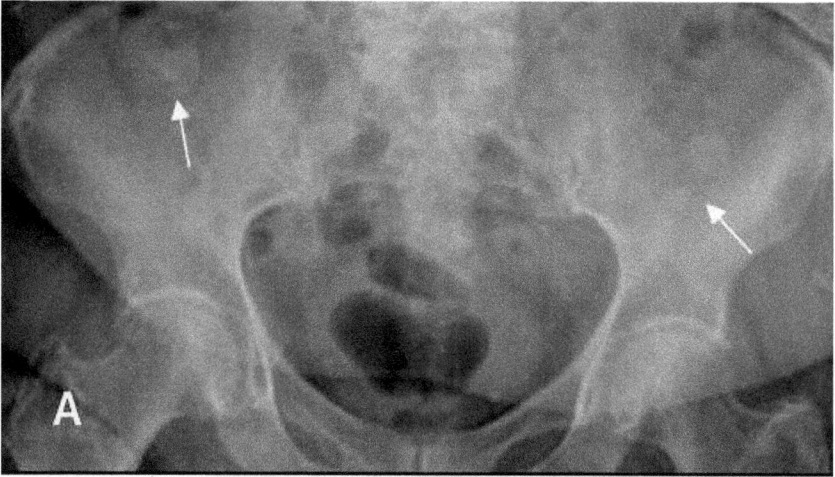

Medication related intramuscular granulomas in the buttocks (white arrows).

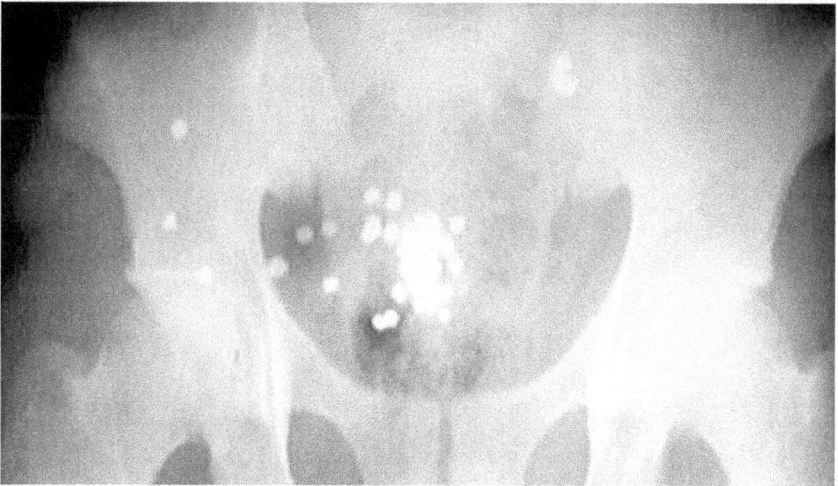

Lead shots.

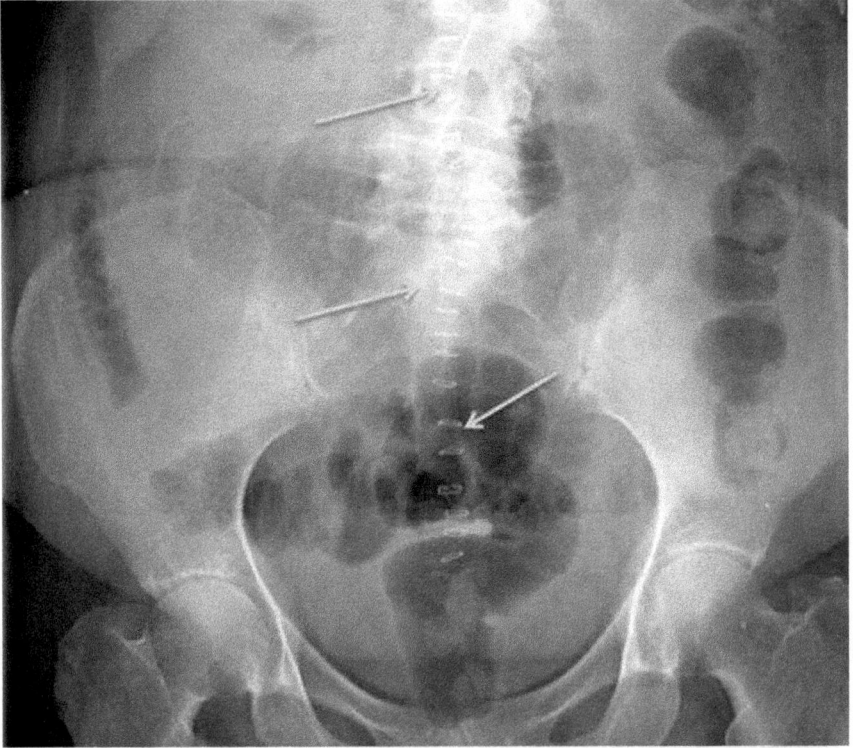

Skin metal clips on a midline incision (white arrows).

2. Medium density or greys in the film:

- Abdominal masses (organs or tumours).
- An accumulation of fluid in the abdominal area (ascites, urine, etc.).
- Colonic displacement by renomegaly.

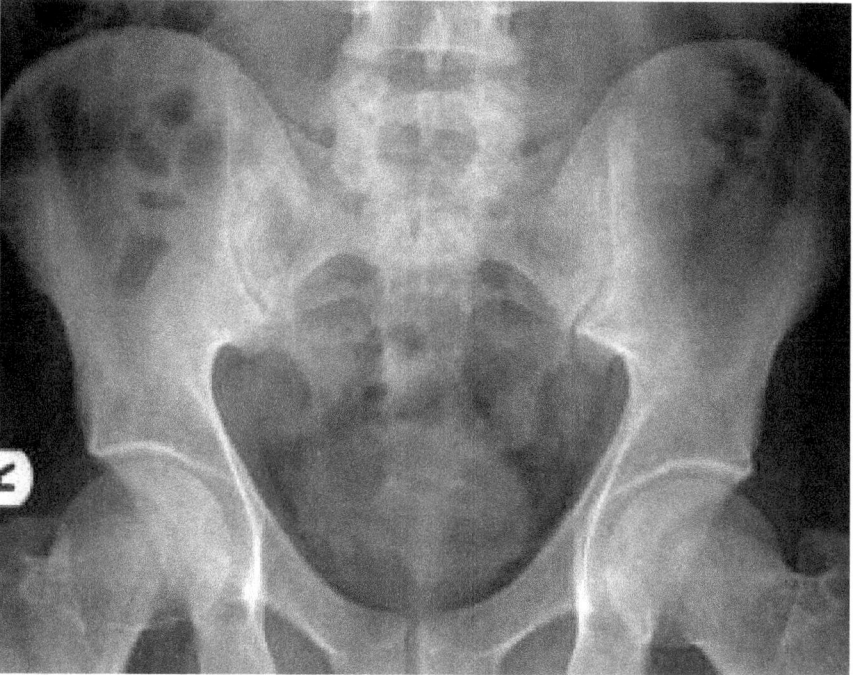

Bladder shadow, density comparable to soft tissue (psoas muscle).

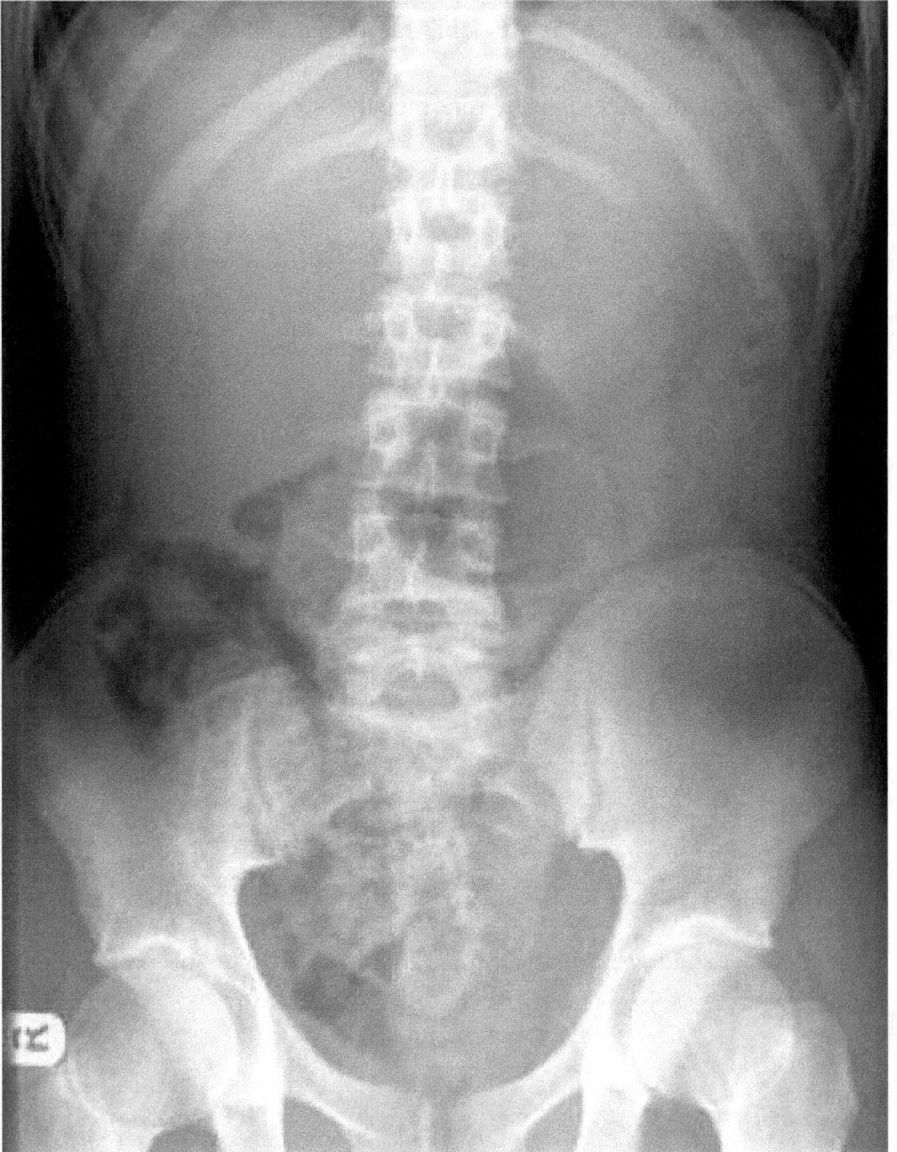

Inferior displacement of the right angle of the colon (gas). Tumour in the right lumbar fossa (RUQ).

3. Low density or darker in the film:

- Pneumo-peritoneum: Perforation of the stomach or intestines (sub diaphragmatic gas).

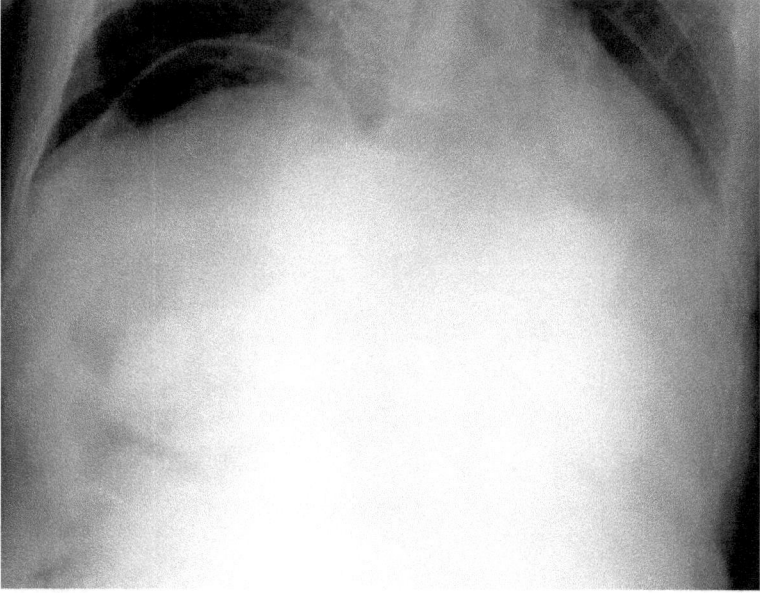

Pneumo-peritoneum, sub diaphragmatic gas.

- Biliary tree gas

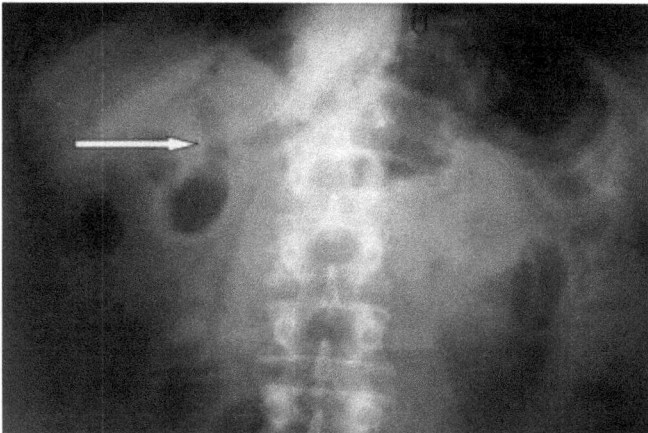

Gas in gallbladder.[32]

- Abdominal abscess.
- Small bowel gas (increased in ileus).
- Retroperitoneal gas.

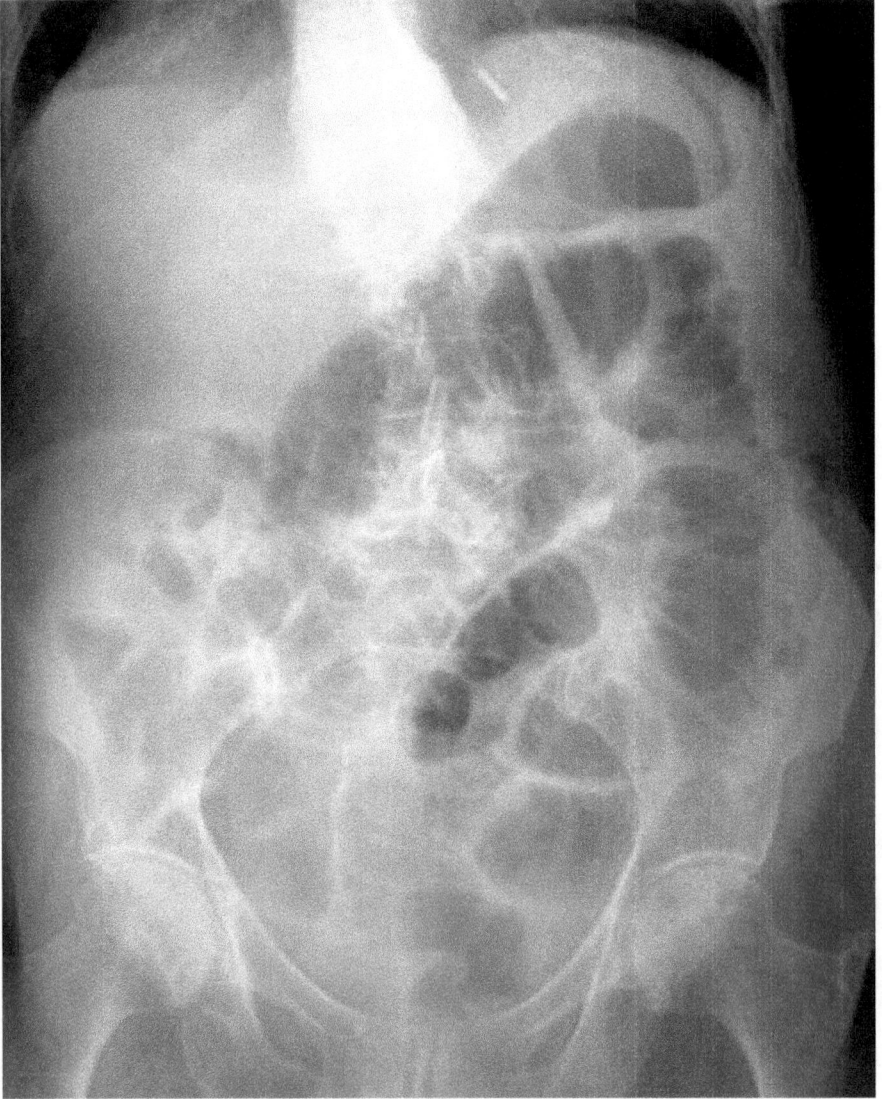

Small bowel gas without levels, patient with potoperative ileus.

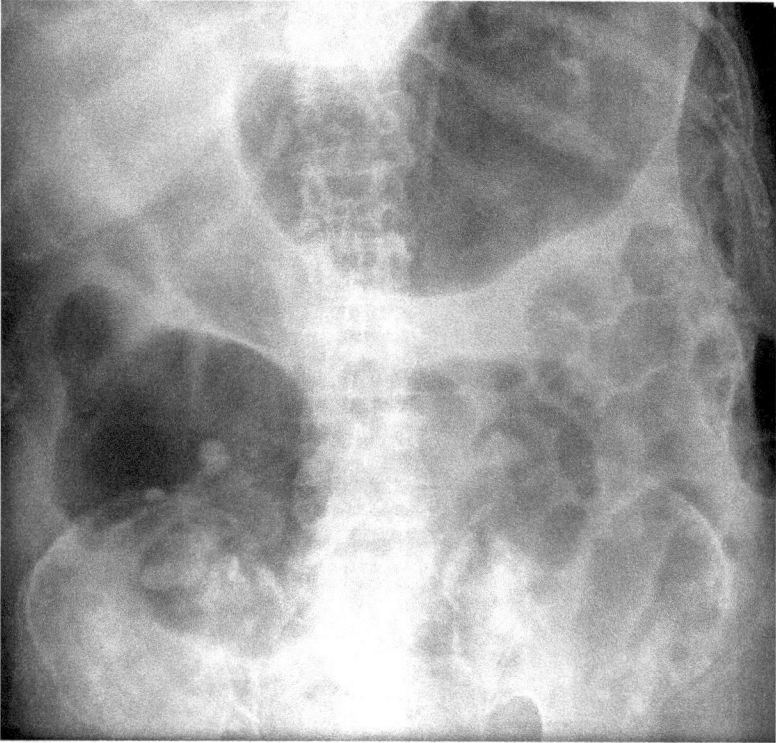

Colon gas without fluid levels and extraurinary abdominal calcifications (bowel).

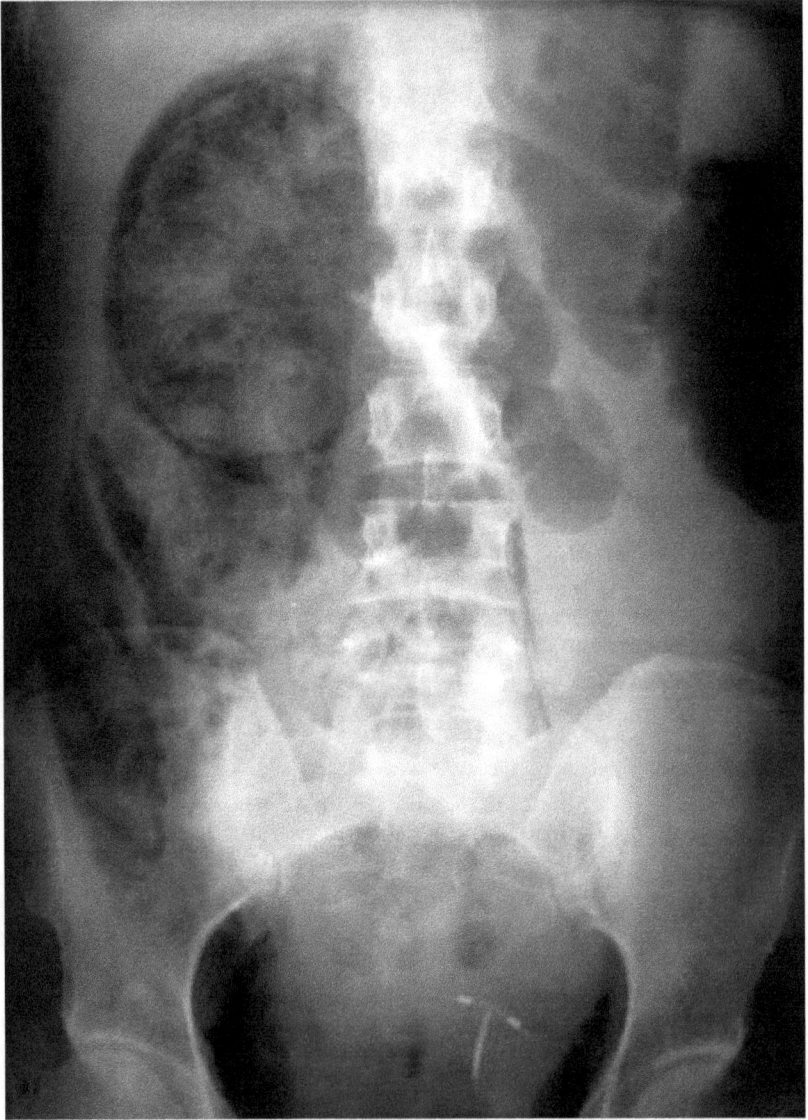

Right kidney emphysematous pyelonephritis.[33]

4. Mixed density:

- Intestinal blockage, with gas/liquid densities levels.

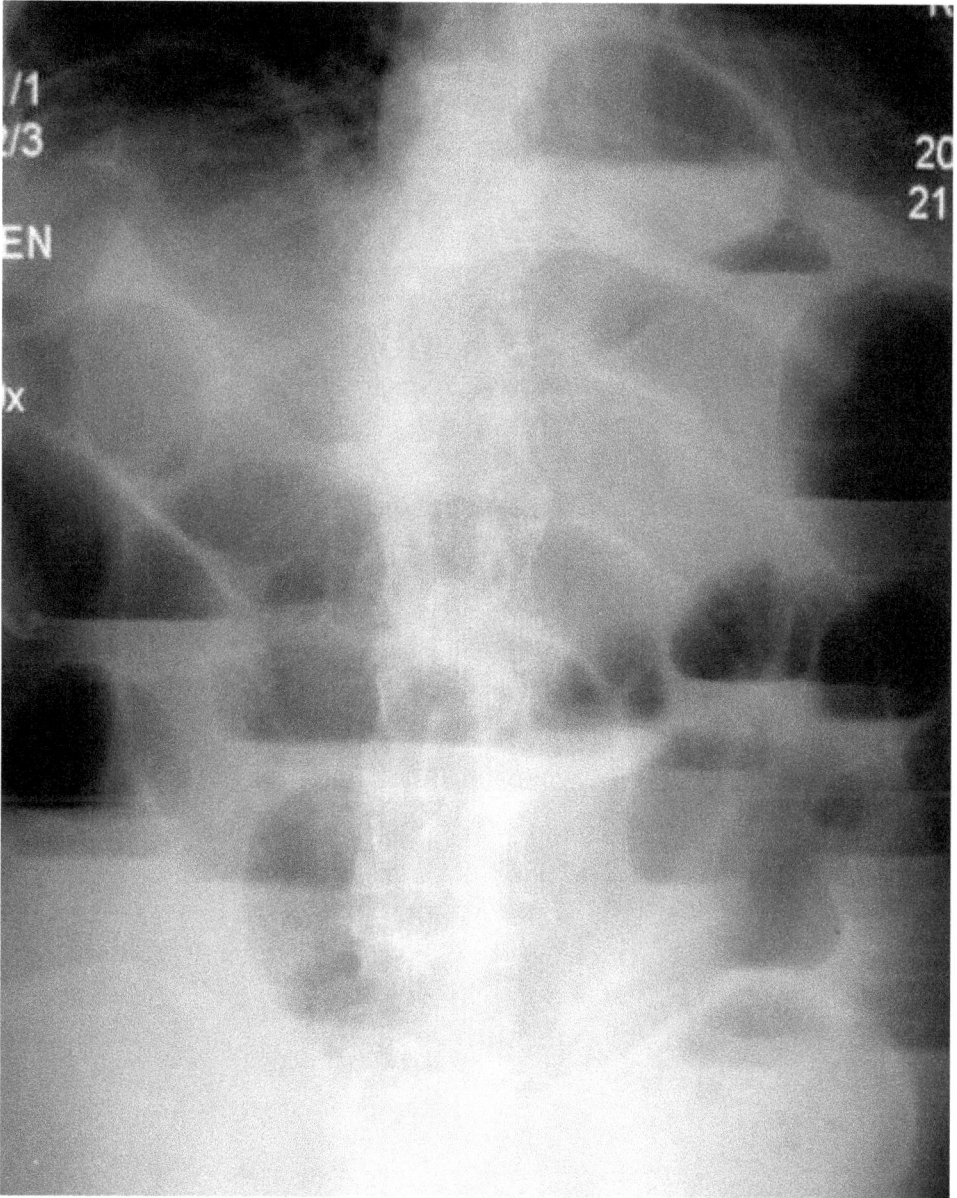

Small bowel obstruction with multiple gas/fluid levels.[34]

CHAPTER 5. CAVEATS.

Factors affecting results:
• Bowel gas, obesity, faeces, fluid, ovarian lesions or calcified uterine fibromas.

• Dye or barium remaining from previous tests.

• During pregnancy the use of ionising radiation should be avoided. If an abdominal X-ray is necessary; the chance of harm to the foetus is usually very small after 8 weeks of gestation.

• Additional points to consider:

a) Children's differences in bone structure.

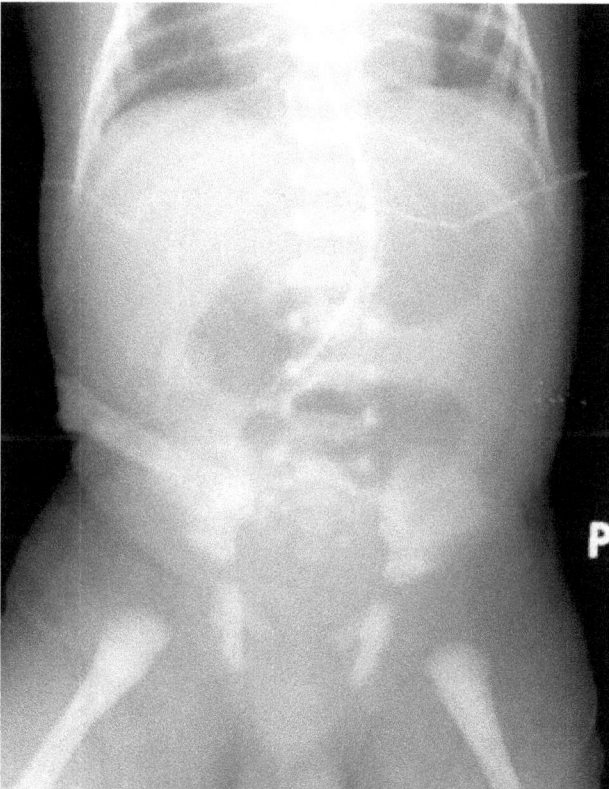

KUB of a newborn child.

b) Congenital anomalies.

Mr J. Clavijo

CHAPTER 6. LATERAL AND OBLIQUE FILMS.

The lateral views are mandatory when a structure is overlying the urinary tract and must be differentiated from (for example) a urinary stone. They are also needed to assess the location of calcifications in the abdomen with respect to the urinary tract.

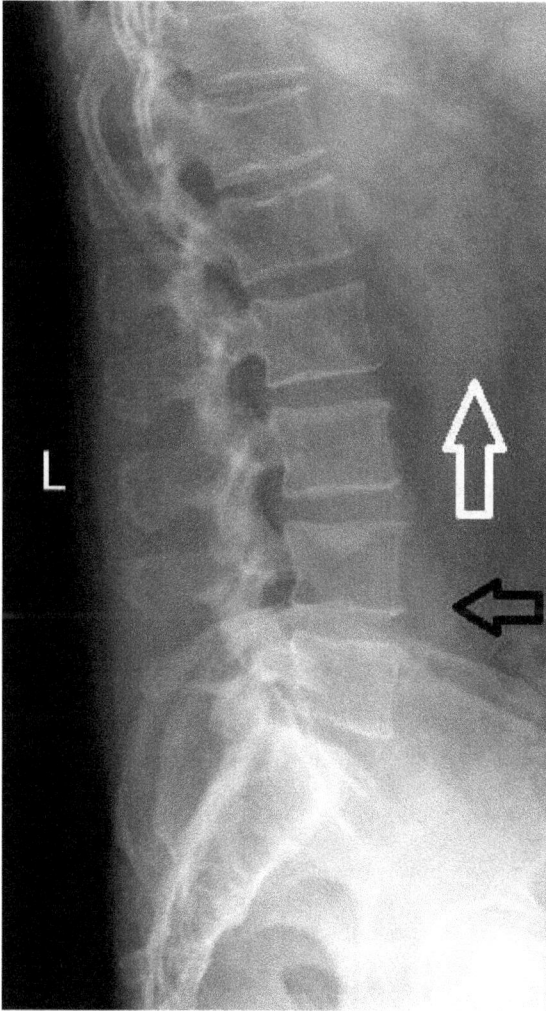

Normal lateral view. Bone structues are clearly seen, as is the psoas (black arrow) and renal area (white arrow).

[7] Liu CW, Tsai TY, Li YF, Lin LC, Wang SJ. Infected primary non-Hodgkin lymphoma of spine. Indian J Orthop 2012; 46:479-82.

[8] Spina bifida occulta am Kreuzbein. www.commons.wikimedia.org. 2014.

[9] From www.commons.wikimedia. 2015.

[10] Pérez Fontes D, Blanco Parra M, Lema Grille J, Toucedo Caamaño V, Novás Castro S, Lamas Cedrón P, Villar Núñez M. Emphysematous cystitis: case report. Arch Esp Urol. 2009 Jun; 62(5):392-5.

[11] de Tarso Machado A; Procópio RJ; Botelho Evangelista F; Dumont Kleinsorge GH; Toledo Afonso C; Pinho NavarroT. Transthoracic retrograde venous bullet embolism: case report and review of the literature. J Vasc Bras. 2008; 7(4):393-396.

[12] Kim JH, Hong JC, Kim MS, Kim SH. Sacral nerve stimulation for treatment of intractable pain associated with cauda equina syndrome. J Korean Neurosurg Soc. 2010 Jun; 47(6):473-6.

[13] Catalano O, Nunziata A, Altei F, Siani A. Suspected ureteral colic: primary helical CT versus selective helical CT after unenhanced radiography and sonography. Am J Roentgenol 2002; 178:379-86.

[14] ACR Appropriateness Criteria for acute onset flank pain, suspicion of stone disease. National Guideline Clearinghouse. www.guidelines.gov. 2005.

[15] Haddad MC, Sharif HS, Abomelha MS, et al. Colour Doppler sonography and plain abdominal radiography in the management of patients with renal colic. Eur Radiol 1994; 4:529-532.

[16] Guidelines for Acute Management of First Presentation of Renal/Ureteric Lithiasis. www.baus.org.uk. 2012.

[17] EAU Guidelines. Urolithiasis. www.uroweb.com. 2014.

[18] Modified from www.hpc.org.ar. 2015.

[19] Schistosomiasis. www.commons.wikimedia.org. 2014.

[20] Case courtesy of Dr Henry Knipe. www.radiopaedia.org. 2015.

[21] From www.wikidoc.org. 2015.

[22] Modified from www.radiologypics.com. 2015.

[23] Case courtesy of Dr Jeremy Jones. www.radiopaedia.org. 2014.

[24] Porcelain gallbladder. www.commons.wikimedia.org. 2014.

[25] Case courtesy of Dr M Osama Yonso. www.radiopaedia.org. 2015.

[26] Bonamigo TP, Erling Jr. N, Salles M. Back pain and infrarenal abdominal aortic aneurysm. J Vasc Br 2004; 3(4):401-2.

[27] From www.ierano.com. 2015.

[28] Case courtesy of Dr Frank Gaillard. www.radiopaedia.org. 2015.

[29] Esmaeili M, Mansouri A, Ghane F. Foreign Body as a Cause of Vaginal Discharge in Childhood. Iranian Journal of Pediatrics, Vol. 18, No. 2, June, 2008, pp. 187-190.

[30] Stravodimos KG, Koritsiadis G, Koutalellis G. Electrical wire as a foreign body in a male urethra: a case report. www.openi.nlm.nih.gov. 2014.

[31] Case courtesy of Dr Hani Salam. www.radiopaedia.org. 2015.

[32] Mohamed A, Bhat N. Gall Stone Ileus: A Rare Complication of Gallstone Disease. Case Report and Literature Review. The Internet Journal of Surgery. 2008 Volume 21 Number 1.

[33] Case courtesy of Dr Mohammad Taghi Niknejad. www.radiopaedia.org. 2015.

[34] Bowel obstruction. www.commons.wikimedia.org. 2014.

AFTERWORD.

When working in Endourology with Graham Watson we found ourselves dealing with significant amounts of KUBs.

The number of interesting and useful findings in KUBs can be as vast as your practice. We then decided to create a tool to help and guide colleagues in the use of this simple and valuable X ray tool.

Neither this book nor any other will give you experience in how to interpret a KUB. We hope this serves you as a guide.

Mr. J. Clavijo Eisele.

Mr J. Clavijo

GLOSSARY.

DGH: District General Hospital.

IUD: Intra Uterine Device.

IVC: Inferior Vena Cava.

IVU: Intra Venous Urography.

KUB: Kidney Ureter Bladder.

LIF: Left Iliac Fossa.

LLQ: Left Lower Quadrant.

LUQ: Left Upper Quadrant.

mAs: milliampers.

NCT: Non-contrast Computer Tomography.

NGT: Naso Gastric Tube.

OA: Ostheo Arthritis.

PE: Pulmonary Embolism.

RIF: Right Iliac Fossa.

RLQ: Right Lower Quadrant.

RUQ: Right Upper Quadrant.

THR: Total Hip Replacement.

USS: Ultrasound scan.

XR: X Ray.

INDEX.

Abdominal XR, 8

Adrenal, 59

Aortic aneurysm, 49

brachitherapy, 44

bullets, 20

calculi. See stones

catheters, 40

cellulitis, 19

Chest XR, 8

coraliform, 32, 33

Eastbourne DGH, iii

foreign bodies, 8, 25

fractures, 12, 16

gangrene, 19, 25

gonadal shield, 10

hernia, 21

Hydatid cyst, 37

ionizing radiation, 8

IUD, 25, 58

IVU, 8, 10, 24

JJ stent, 8, 32, 40, 41

KUB, i, 2, 4, 8, 10, 25, 29, 70, 76

metastasis, 12, 13, 14

nephrocalcinosis, 39

Nephrostomy, 40

Non-contrast computed tomography, 29

occlusion, 24

osteoblastic, 12, 13, 14, 16

osteolythic, 12

Paget's disease, 16, 17

pelvic kidney, 24, 41

penile prosthesis, 21, 46

Phleboliths, 53

pneumoperitoneum, 11

Pneumo-peritoneum, 64

pregnancy, 36, 70

Prostate, 39, 44

Psoas, 19

pyelonephritis, 24, 25, 67

rem, 8

renal artery, 50

Renal colic, 8

renal pelvis, 24, 26, 32, 34, 40

retroperitoneal, 19

Sacral nerve stimulator, 20

Schistosomiasis, 38, 73

scoliosis, 14, 15

spina bifida, 16

Steinstrasse, 35

stones, 8, 9, 25, 29, 33, 34, 39, 51, 53

technique, 9, 10

THR, 17

Ultrasound scan, 29

urinary extravasation, 11

urinary sphincter, 45

urostomy, 20

X rays, 8

www.ingramcontent.com/pod-product-compliance
Lightning Source LLC
Chambersburg PA
CBHW071117210326
41519CB00020B/6332